# A MARKETER'S GUIDE TO PHYSICIAN RELATIONS

## BEST PRACTICES FOR SUCCESSFUL SALES PROGRAMS

### KRISS BARLOW, RN, MBA

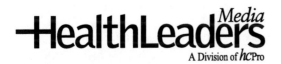

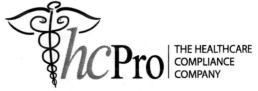

THE HEALTHCARE
COMPLIANCE
COMPANY

*A Marketer's Guide to Physician Relations: Best Practies for Successful Sales Programs* is published by HCPro, Inc.

Copyright © 2007 HCPro, Inc.

ISBN: 978-1-60146-074-5

HCPro, Inc., provides information resources for the healthcare industry.

HCPro, Inc., is not affiliated in any way with The Joint Commission, which owns the JCAHO and Joint Commission trademarks.

Kriss Barlow, RN, MBA, Author
Gienna Shaw, Editor
Amy Anthony, Executive Editor
Matthew Cann, Group Publisher
Mike Mirabello, Senior Graphic Artist
Michael Roberto, Layout Artist
Doug Ponte, Cover Designer

Matthew Kuhrt, Copyeditor
Lauren Rubenzahl, Proofreader
Susan Darbyshire, Art Director
Darren Kelly, Books Production Supervisor
Claire Cloutier, Production Manager
Jean St. Pierre, Director of Operations

Advice given is general. Readers should consult professional counsel for specific legal, ethical, or clinical questions. Arrangements can be made for quantity discounts. For more information, contact:

HCPro, Inc.
P.O. Box 1168
Marblehead, MA 01945
Telephone: 800/650-6787 or 781/639-1872
Fax: 781/639-2982
E-mail: *customerservice@hcpro.com*

**HCPro, Inc., is the parent company of Healthleaders Media.**
**Visit HCPro at its World Wide Web sites:**
*www.healthleadersmedia.com, www.hcpro.com*, and *www.hcmarketplace.com*

Rev. 11/2007
21292

# Contents

  **A Marketer's Guide to Physician Relations**

**A Marketer's Guide to Physician Relations**

# Acknowledgments

With all the energy and interest in physician relations, and the encouragement from the excellent editorial team at HealthLeaders Media, the timing seemed right to talk about the people and practices that make it work.

Credit needs to be given to the great clients and industry experts who found time to share their insights. Working on a tight schedule, they found time in their already busy lives to provide insights and real, in-the-trenches advice. I am grateful and salute their efforts; they are the innovators who make this industry proud.

Relationships with physicians or colleagues work best when they are founded on trust. Allison McCarthy, trusted and talented cofounder of Barlow/McCarthy, deserves extra special recognition for her unconditional willingness to support me with this effort and to share timely words of wisdom. Her attention to detail and real-life experiences are vital difference-makers in the market. Dave Zirkle, our consulting partner, was the man of the hour. He provided fabulous support to the clients and to the book's efforts. I'm so proud of our team—consummate professionals who have the clients' needs front and center.

And on a personal note, I believe happy people take on more, connect in more meaningful ways, and contribute more in all walks of life. At the center of my world are the greatest contributors to my happiness: my husband, Doug; our fabulous boys Tony, Jon, and Greg; and our daughter-in-law, Ingrid. They love me, support me, and give me the energy for life. And life is good!

# About the author

## Kriss Barlow, RN, MBA

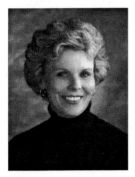

**Kriss Barlow, RN, MBA,** has spent her entire professional career—more than 25 years—in the healthcare industry. Even at an early age, through the eyes of her father, a doctor, she was witness to hospital-physician relationships and the tug of different worlds trying to share solutions that would benefit the patient.

Kriss, who holds a bachelor's degree in nursing from Augustana College and a master's degree in business administration from the University of Nebraska, has spent the past 11 years sharing her extensive knowledge of clinical and business development with clients, helping them with physician relations, retention, sales, physician recruitment, and medical staff development. Today, she is principal of Barlow/McCarthy, a consulting group focused on hospital-physician solutions. She focuses on strategy, medical staff planning, and relationship models. Her business partner, Allison McCarthy, is a former client who specializes in physician recruitment and tracking. At the end of the day, her client relationships and the opportunity to help them achieve success are the most fulfilling aspects of her job.

While her clinical background helps in her current role, strategy, program development, and business solutions are her real passion. A recognized expert in these areas, Kriss is a frequent speaker whose presentations are informed by her vast experience and made more lively by her many stories from the trenches. She has presented at the Forum for Healthcare Strategists, the Society for Healthcare Strategy and Market Development of the American Hospital Association, the Healthcare Financial Management Association, and the American College of Healthcare Executives and is a regular speaker for HealthLeaders Media's Webcasts on strategic marketing and physician relations. She is a faculty member for the American Academy of Medical Management's Physician Recruitment program and serves on the Board of Directors for the National Medical Staff Certification program. She is also a certified sales instructor.

Kriss is the co-author of a previous book, *Physician Relations Today: A Model for Growth* and was a contributing author to another book, *The Business of Medical Practice*. She writes a regular column on physician sales and relations for *Healthcare Strategic Management*, a monthly newsletter published by HealthLeaders Media.

When Kriss isn't taking care of her clients, she's busy with her family. Her husband, Doug, is the steadying force in her life and her biggest supporter. Together, they have three fabulous sons and one charming daughter-in-law. With one of her "boys" ready to begin a residency in orthopedics, the cycle or medical staff relationships and expectations, she notes, is set to begin again.

# Introduction

## Physician relations programs: Why now?

Creating or enhancing physician relations programs is very much in vogue
these days. The increasing number of healthcare options, shrinking profit
margins, and more competition is driving this trend. The current heavy
emphasis on working more closely with physicians to earn referral opportunities is fueled by the recognition that, while consumers are becoming more
and more proactive when making decisions about their own healthcare, the
physician is still a pivotal decision-maker when it comes to determining where
a patient is admitted or where a procedure is performed.

Meanwhile, physicians are going through significant challenges of their own.
The practice of medicine and the economics of the profession have changed;
days of entrepreneurial solo practitioners are all but gone for the new physician. There's a disconnect within the ranks as maturing physicians struggle to
understand the needs and wants of their young colleagues. They're working
harder and netting less income. Practice viability is front and center for them.

As we discuss how to grow referrals and encourage physician relationships
and loyalty with our organization or group, we have to begin in their
world. Physicians aren't gleeful, and they're not looking for gleeful partners.

Understanding things from the perspective of today's physicians is essential before an organization can employ any of the best practices for physician relations programs that are described in this book.

> *"There is nothing easy about managing today's health-care organization. The market challenges are abundant. At the center is the patient and his or her physician. We must find ways to create meaningful relationships with our doctors at every level," "Successful sales programs depend upon a positive attitude and a new way of strategic thinking by hospital administrators."*
>
> — Tom May, president of HCA's Far West Division in Henderson, NV

## What best practices do

For more than a decade, I have been blessed with the opportunity to work as a consultant in physician relations with some of the best people and the finest organizations in the country. Working with these organizations to develop their models has given me unique insight into the inner workings and the must-have best practices that lead to success. Time has a marvelous way of weeding through the shiny glow of newness and exposing us to those attributes that, when sustained, really do make a difference. The best practices described in this book are just that—time-tested attributes that are present when programs sustain and continue to deliver measurable results.

The best programs are focused on building relationships through regular, face-to-face visits between representatives and referring physicians. It's that simple—sort of. To earn new referrals, it's not enough to know what the physicians need. You must also recognize that the business we want currently goes somewhere else. For representatives to earn those referrals away from the competition, they must do more than just tell the physicians what their organization has to offer. Best-practice organizations position their differences, gain the physicians' trust, and earn the opportunity to care for the referred patients.

Facilities across the country have hired representatives to call on physicians and encourage new referrals. Some have carefully groomed the representatives and selected a special group of physicians for them to target. Others have said, "We hired someone and turned him/her loose to make this happen." As the programs, process, and measures are evaluated, there are some central themes that appear in those organizations that are seeing the best results. Those hospitals and group practices that are gaining momentum by enhancing relationships with key physicians are able to sustain those relationships and achieve mutual benefit.

> "*If we are going to ask leaders to be effective in developing a physician sales function, we need to clearly articulate the vision and then provide them with the right support and resources to make it happen. This is an area where you do get what you pay for.*"
>
> — Tom May, president of HCA's Far West Division in Henderson, NV

# Best-practice magic

This book does not contain any magical formulas or phrases. Most of the best practices are foundational elements. Sometimes they seem so simple they are assumed. Sometimes they are recognized at the onset but then become too hard to implement because of internal turf wars or politics. The reality is that it is often the little things that can make a difference—and give us the edge when much of the choice is very subjective.

Truth be told, almost nobody has all the best practices in place all the time. Maybe that's the reality of anything that is relationship driven. But programs across the country have continued to demonstrate excellence in one or several areas, and they are worth learning more about.

Hospitals, large group practices, freestanding services, and other organizations are constantly on the prowl for more effective techniques to garner new business. This book and the best practices described in it give you the chance to size up what you have and help you determine whether there are areas where you may need to focus a bit more attention.

I focused on attributes that play out in every environment. If you are an academic medical center, there will certainly be unique best-practice attributes that are essential for your survival that may not be relevant for a rural community medical center and vice versa. Maybe you will have one or two other best-practice strategies that you find especially important for your type of delivery system.

**A Marketer's Guide to Physician Relations**

With the attention earned from sustained growth in referral volumes comes the expansion of the sales effort we currently know and use. While the book highlights a couple of areas that I envision to be future difference-makers, physician relations representatives and their leaders are certainly among the most innovative people within healthcare systems. More new and different strategies to earn the referrals are certain to be discovered, which is what I love most about this field and the people: The passion, the fortitude to try new things in an environment that does not really love change, and the never-ending drive to make a difference.

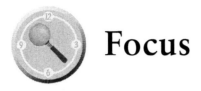

# Focus

## Focus on goals, roles, and expectations

The best physician relations programs generally start with a clear sense of direction. When a hospital or health system begins a program with clear goals and expectations, it is easier to maintain focus as the years go by. Here's the thing: Nobody ever intentionally takes a program off course. The most difficult aspect of focus (and the reason it earns the number-one slot among all eight best practices) is that it is lost in bits and pieces. A must-attend meeting or a series of meetings robs us of an hour here and an hour there. We launch one little project that we swear will last only a week or two. We agree to help out with the board president's pet project just this one time. The next thing you know, we're bogged down in the quagmire of hours and details and tasks that each of these small distractions require. The meetings and the extra projects might seem like a good use of our time at the moment we start them, but cumulatively, they have a way of pulling the physician relations program off course.

Maintaining focus is like sticking to a diet. You don't gain 10 pounds by eating one candy bar. Rather, it's having just a little bite of chocolate after supper each night, going out to dinner and splurging just that one time, and eating a piece of birthday cake and some ice cream to celebrate a special occasion. It's insidious. Successful dieters—and successful physician relations program leaders—know that they must recognize those areas where they are vulnerable, create mechanisms for accountability, and make certain that everyone is on the same page. Otherwise, your diet—or your physician relations program—will slip.

"The bottom line for keeping people focused is not getting caught up in specialty projects, trends, or trying to be all things to all people," says Mike Riley, vice president (VP) of sales for HCA Continental Division in Denver. "It's easy to get caught up in that, but what we have learned is that the more we stick to what we were hired to do—looking at who we are targeting, assessing their potential financial contribution, and making sure we focus on spending time with them—the more we deliver real results to the organization."

For best-practice organizations, focus is evident in all four key areas:

1. Program goals

2. The role of the field representative

3. Marketplace challenges and opportunities

4. Long-range vision and goals

**A Marketer's Guide to Physician Relations**

> *"It's a big circle, and you've got to have all the balls balanced at one time."*

— Don Fischer, director of business development, *Southeast Missouri Hospital*

## Focus on program goals

The enthusiasm and energy exhibited by teams as they embark on a focused physician relationship strategy is awesome. Internal stakeholders, especially those who have worked hard to get a physician relations representative on board, have high expectations for the new representative. When I talk to leadership and operational teams that are in the process of developing a physician relations program, I often ask about their expectations for the program. Everyone recognizes that the representative's job is to grow referrals. But when it comes to setting priorities and taking action to actually make this happen, the conversation quickly turns to what the representative is going to do for each individual and his or her service area. And guess what? Everyone has a different expectation. Each person sees the sales effort from his or her own perspective. Everyone has great ideas about how the program will help grow business. But no one has really talked much about this internally because each person assumes that everyone else is on the same page.

### Create an internal communications plan

So how do you manage these varied expectations and ensure consistent focus? First, you have to put it into the right perspective. "When you look at a referral strategy, the whole thing is a game of inches," says Michael Thomas,

VP of strategic planning and marketing at East Texas Medical Center Regional Healthcare System in Tyler. "We can't just describe a vision and hope that it happens. We have to develop a tactical approach that will deliver results and ensure that everyone is on board."

The best approach is to create a formal physician strategy plan that details who will deal with each segment of the medical staff. This not only aligns the objectives and manages the overlap but also provides a visual depiction of the activity level for each segment.

Here are some steps you can take to improve internal communications and help maintain focus for the program:

- Meet with internal stakeholders to agree on the focus of the program. Summarize the discussion in writing, and distribute this document to the entire team to get final consensus. The group may decide on a focus for the first three to six months of the program, after which the team can be reconvened to assess results and determine whether changes should be made.

- Design the tactics and targets based on the agreed-upon focus. Again, this should be shared in a document with the team so that any specific service deliverables or physician targets that team members have in mind are documented.

**A Marketer's Guide to Physician Relations**

- Provide regular reports on tactical accomplishments and feedback on results to the team. These could consist of weekly e-mail briefs and/or monthly activity reports with market intelligence and summaries of referral barriers. The sales staff will want to provide the team with planned actions as a result of these findings so they're aware of how the team plans to integrate these findings into their referral growth strategy.

- Conduct evaluation meetings with the team on a regular basis (e.g., every 90 days) to review the original objectives, field findings, and new business outcomes. Adjust the plan as appropriate, making sure to get consensus from the team at each interval.

You're probably thinking this can be done informally. I recommend against this, however. Although an informal approach might work at the onset, even the most dedicated people find it hard to do all they should (and keep doing it) if there is no formal system of accountability. Also, over time, as changes occur in staffing and priorities, the internal communication plan is an excellent way to keep your physician strategy front and center for those who need to implement it. That's what makes it a best practice.

### Explain sales to internal stakeholders

To set a clear direction for your physician relations program, you must also have an understanding about what sales is versus what it is not. Understand what it is *supposed* to accomplish versus what it *could* do. And share this information with your internal stakeholders. The best plan in the world won't improve the focus of your program if your internal audience doesn't understand the sales process—and what it takes to get new business from physicians.

To keep a program on task, internal stakeholders must understand the process of earning new referrals. I am not suggesting that every leader in the organization must understand every nuance of sales or even that they must completely embrace the concept. What I am saying, however, is that people who have oversight for the physician relations program must regularly remind leaders of the need to keep the sales representatives focused on their tasks. You must understand the typical hospital leader's perception of sales and help him or her to understand what it really takes out in the field to grow the organization's business.

Many internal stakeholders do not really understand growth. They may think the physician sales representative's role is to learn what the physicians feel is wrong with the organization or to increase satisfaction among loyal physicians. They are not aware that there is a difference between taking care of those who already send you referrals and increasing referrals from doctors who have little or no loyalty to your facility. The latter, of course, is key to growth. If a physician raises a concern, the organization must listen and respond to it.

Fixing that issue, by the way, does not ensure referral growth. Rather, it provides the chance to keep referrals we otherwise may have lost and continue earning the business we already have. This approach can earn the representative favor in the eyes of the physician. The ability to listen and respond is a key element of the role, but the focus of a growth strategy is finding ways to get new business by using positive messages to engage in a dialogue about their needs and then offering the organization's services to meet those needs. This is the understanding that must be established for sales in order to maintain focus.

One of the jobs of the physician relations representative is to respond to physicians' needs. The doctor says something must be fixed, and the representative deals with it. Many incorrectly perceive that as sales. In fact, selling is more about *discovering* physicians' needs. The representative wants the doctor to change his or her referral patterns. The physician is resistant to change. This type of relationship building requires attentiveness to the unique nuances of how each physician practices and an ability to listen for those nuggets of information that provide the salesperson with an opening to convince the physician to change his or her referral pattern. Although making operational changes encourages those who are on the medical staff to feel listened to and appreciated, tangible actions (e.g., ordering a new piece of equipment, changing a rule, or adapting a schedule) are also necessary to keep the business you already receive. That's not sales—it's maintenance.

Contrast this with a situation wherein the physician has no relationship or a limited relationship with your facility. Although your loyal physicians may see a certain service or benefit as a given or as a value-added option, a physician who does not currently make referrals to your facility may see the service or benefit as a new opportunity. In the world of sales, we call that a *gift*. Why? Because most healthcare facilities aren't that different from one another. For the most part, they share pretty much the same features. It is the subtle differences—the quality of the person delivering the service, the way in which the service is delivered, or the way in which clinical outcomes are reported— that can convince a physician to change his or her referral patterns.

The sales representative must uncover these nuances. The sales rep must probe to see whether the facility offers something that is truly different from the competition and then encourage the physician to try it out and determine whether the experience warrants a change. The challenge is to keep the sales effort focused on activities that truly bring in new business. Anything that distracts or dilutes your efforts can make you lose focus. A key to successful relationship-selling with long-term value is the ability to be consistent. A consistent message, approach, style, and regularity of meetings all make the difference.

Columbus (OH) Children's Hospital has had a physician relations program in place for nearly 10 years. It is led by Donna Teach, VP of market development and promotion. Her approach is to look at the objectives for a specific target audience and then create strategies and tactics around how the target audience wants to build a relationship with the hospital. "We have our programs built with an outside-in look. Our focus is predicated on the needs of our referring physicians and how they want to have a relationship with the institution, versus the other way around," she says. Once her team has developed the strategy and determined the tactical approach, they streamline the communication channels so that the entire organization is focused on consistent messages.

 **A Marketer's Guide to Physician Relations**

# Focus on the role of the field representative

To maintain a focused physician relations program, a proactive field effort must be the focal point of the program. That means the representative goes to the practices of those physicians who have the potential to bring more business your way. At the heart of the interaction is shared communication and dialogue with the physician. Best-practice programs detail the number of visits and other relationship-enhancing activities that they expect the sales representative to accomplish. They focus on specific services that are ready for growth, target physicians who are likely to refer patients to those services, and make certain that the representative understands the areas in which they have true market differentiation. Finally, they train the representative to create the right dialogue to uncover the right referral opportunities. To keep the representative focused on creating referral opportunities in the field, consider the following:

- Despite the pace and demand of field visits, many organizations expect their salespeople to develop a business strategy and create business plans. Although it's true that most salespeople are also capable of sales planning, almost none have the right background to create a comprehensive physician business plan. If you want a solid and efficiently prepared plan, then get someone who knows hospital data to support the plan development, use data to finalize the target lists, and then let the salespeople work on it.

- Successful organizations create a solid strategy for service lines that the organization has targeted for increased business. Ensure that these services are ready for new business and that service line leaders are ready to support the sales team, as needed, with messaging, physician-friendly service, and time in the field.

- It's also a good idea to create an internal mechanism for issue resolution so that the representative can easily forward physician concerns to those with operational responsibility and be assured that they will manage the resolution and communicate the outcome with both the physician and the representative.

- The representatives could be great helpers for countless other activities, but that's the not the real reason you hired them. Authentic commitment to growing referrals means a single-mindedness and concentration in the field. The vulnerability is that since they are "can-do" people, there's a tremendous temptation to use them for other tasks that they can do well but for which they were not hired.

You might be wondering why it's so important to differentiate between fieldwork and other work of the physician relations program. If you are thinking about assigning additional tasks to representatives, first make sure you can answer "yes" to the following questions:

- Is the task related to the physicians the representative is targeted to visit?

- Will the relationship between the representative and the physician advance as a result of the activity?

- Can we expect to gain new referrals as a result of the effort?

Resist the temptation to answer the questions with a qualified yes, even if it seems like the task might help accomplish the goals indirectly. Time after time, I have seen programs that started with a very clear field focus falter because of a little thing here and a little thing there. Next thing you know, the representatives aren't doing all of that crucial fieldwork you hoped for when you hired them in the first place.

## Keep field representatives in the field

Best-practice organizations are cognizant of internal workflow. Other health-care workers can multitask. They work on many different projects, they perform many different tasks, and their schedules are flexible. Further, they can easily stop what they're doing to attend a meeting and then pick up right where they left off when it's done. Field-focused representatives, however, simply cannot work this way. Every time they are called into the office, they lose valuable field time. If there is a meeting on campus at 1 p.m., for example, the representative likely loses at least two appointments that day because of the time needed to travel to campus, attend the meeting, and then travel back into the field again.

Focusing first and foremost on sales means that we create an environment that requires and allows the representative to be in the field. At a practical level, this means making choices about which meetings are critical for representatives to attend.

Representatives are usually asked to contribute to meetings beginning at about the three-month mark. This is good news and bad news. The good news is that leaders and other stakeholders are showing an interest in the success of the program. They want to know what the representative is hearing and learning in the field. There is a level of excitement and anticipation as new physicians appear in the hall and the departments and services start seeing increased referrals. Representatives are invited to share what they've learned at service-line meetings, with the marketing and business development staff, and at medical staff and section meetings. When you think about all the possible meetings in one week at your organization, however, you discover the bad news. If the representative is in meetings, he or she is not in the field. Best-practice organizations manage this dilemma in several ways:

- They decide which meetings really count and encourage representatives to attend when they feel it is necessary

- They use quality reports and outcomes to demonstrate the program's impact, instead of having representatives report to internal stakeholders during a presentation

- They appoint a sales team leader as the liaison for internal meetings

**A Marketer's Guide to Physician Relations**

- They schedule meetings on Monday mornings or Friday afternoons, when field productivity tends to drop

### Foster a culture that supports growth

Best-practice organizations are focused on generating new business. In fact, they often have one or more representatives who are focused solely on generating new business. But these organizations also recognize that one or two people can't do it all by themselves. Everyone in the organization must pull together to help position services to earn new referrals.

The culture of these best-practice organizations is oriented to growth. Of course, culture is deeply ingrained at most healthcare facilities. It can't be changed overnight. But there are real benchmarks that indicate a strong orientation toward the physician's role in bringing referrals to the facility and the representative's role in making that happen. A growth- or sales-oriented culture is one in which the internal stakeholders recognize and value the contributions of those customers—especially physicians—who bring business in the door. Best-practice organizations have a culture that embodies the value of sales. For example:

- They value the role of each physician who brings patients to the facility for care.

- They understand the impact of hospitalist admissions and that the ease of maintaining primary care relationships with the primary care physicians (PCP) is gone. Finding new ways to connect and relate with PCPs is essential.

- They consistently deliver on basic expectations. Physician relations programs are obligated to promise only what the organization can actually deliver. The internal clinical and operational staff must fulfill those basic promises.

- They realize that communication among clinicians, representatives, referring physicians, and leaders is crucial. This is true whether the news is good or bad, whether standards are not met, or when there are victories to celebrate. The representative and the internal stakeholders work hard to communicate changes, so there is real-time knowledge of happenings.

Organizations with a growth or sales culture also recognize that once the internal strategic decision is made to grow a service line, there must be consistent ability to meet that need. We can't ask a representative to grow business at a certain number per day or only on certain days when volumes are down. When an organization decides to grow a service line and asks referring physicians to send the organization new business, the organization had better be able to accommodate those patients. If you ask for new business, you have an obligation to do everything in your power to accept it.

For some organizations, this means they must reassess their payer strategy so that those practices targeted for more referrals can send all patients to the same referral source. For others, they must create access lines to streamline the transport. Still others have created additional triage functions to support the referring physician (this has been expedited with the augmented use of

**A Marketer's Guide to Physician Relations**

hospitalists). Organizations with a focused sales culture encourage, embrace, and welcome new business.

# Focus on marketplace challenges and opportunities

No discussion of focus can be complete without highlighting the positive impact of a program that is focused on growing the right business. At Memorial Health University Medical Center, Inc., in Savannah, GA, Don E. Tomberlin, Sr. VP of regional development and sales, has fine-tuned in such a way that he can succinctly and consistently describe his focus and the reasons for it as often as is needed to keep focused on the right targets.

"We've identified three categories of the medical staff," he says. "Those we consider loyal are those who are giving 80% or more of their business to us. Those who are splitters are those who give us between 20% and 79% of their inpatient business. We have determined that we can change maybe 30%–40% of that splitter business when they start at that level. But those physicians who send us any less than 20% at the outset of our efforts we have determined we cannot change and do not justify the additional expense."

Best-practice organizations target the right services and the right physicians to grow their referrals.

## Gain internal agreement on the approach

Most programs have, in response to the needs of the referring physician, worked to provide a single contact to act as a central resource on acute care services within the organization. He or she is the central resource for the target physician on all the organization's services. This tactic positions that person to communicate on behalf of the entire organization and to reach out to the appropriate clinical expert when the need arises, rather than sending out multiple people to pitch one product each. What a wise thing to do! The challenge, however, is determining which services to highlight. This is where focus really comes into play. Every service wants to have its attributes front and center. And this is complicated by the fact that they do not clearly understand how sales works and that bringing in new referrals takes more than making a onetime pitch.

The first step is to make a list of the service lines that are key to your facility's growth strategy. The following questions will help narrow the list to the top three or four spotlight services:

1. **Is there good upside potential?** The right service is one that has solid revenue and volume potential. Time with physicians is precious, and the face-to-face approach to earning business is expensive. At the end of the day, the physician relations program has an obligation to ensure profitability. "We identify the service lines we believe we want to focus on and then identify the current referral patterns," explains Sue Pietrafeso, director of outreach programs at Sunrise Health Systems in Las Vegas. "We then determine what the natural growth is for that clinical area and what we believe we can redirect from competitors. We then project what we think we can move, and if we don't believe we can move enough to make it worthwhile, then we remove that service area from

 **A Marketer's Guide to Physician Relations**

our targets. But if we believe there is potential, we forecast the actual growth we expect we can achieve and then keep track of what is actually happening so we can then measure the effectiveness of the strategy."

2. **Do you have capacity?** Internal capacity includes not only the number of beds but also the capability of support services or other departments that are critical for throughput. For example, is there room in the surgery schedule? Can you get MRIs done in a timely fashion? Capacity means that you have the clinical, nursing, and technical staff to ensure that all patients can be treated if new referrals are generated. Capacity also refers to specialists. You must have an adequate number of specialists who are interested in increasing their patient base. As you evaluate this aspect of capacity, make sure that you have access to specialists who accept the type of patients that you anticipate attracting. Pay attention to the payer expectations or the level of workup required. Growing "select referrals" can be done, but it requires a very different model and method. Specialist capacity also means that the specialists will value the new business and treat the referring physicians in a way that encourages them to use your specialists rather than the competition's. Keep politics in mind if you have several specialty groups all vying for these new referrals. Again, it is about preplanning, strong internal communication, and, of course, focus.

3. **Can you differentiate?** Another area to evaluate when you are determining which areas to position for growth is your ability to differentiate your service from the one that the referring physician currently uses. In

today's environment, the referrals you want are generally already being served by another provider. If you are going to ask a physician to shift his or her referrals, the representative had better be able to draw a clear distinction between you and your competitors. We'll discuss differentiation later in the book.

4. **Is there market appeal?** The right services are also those that have appeal in the marketplace. Often, the motivation for selecting services is driven exclusively by margins. But this isn't always the best approach. Recently, I was talking to a hospital leader about his targeted areas for growth. "We're very interested in growing our outpatient radiology business," he said. "We have all the equipment, and the margins are excellent." This made great sense to me, until I had a conversation with another member of the leadership team. "The margins *are* great," he told me with a laugh. "But there are three freestanding facilities within half a mile of our campus. They are lovely, accommodating, and have physician investors. Our facility is in the basement, has no streamlined access for outpatients, and is only open from 8 a.m. to 5 p.m." Remember: You can sell only what someone wants to buy.

## *Target the right physicians*

Assuming you know what to position, your next area is to determine which physicians can send that type of referral your way. If your focus is on retaining business, you have it easy—you simply target those who are currently sending you the bulk of their referrals. But what if you want to grow business? There are several criteria to help you identify the right targets for referral growth:

**A Marketer's Guide to Physician Relations**

1. **Opportunity.** Target physicians who have a practice mix that allows them to send more referrals your way. When creating the business plan, determine which physicians split their referrals among facilities.

2. **Ability.** Make sure that there are no precluding circumstances (e.g., payer mix or patient preference) that would have an impact on your ability to encourage the physician to send more of those referrals to you.

3. **Specialty.** Include both specialists and PCPs in the targeted group. If you want to grow certain clinical areas, you must assess the type of specialist who would refer for that service and evaluate how patients end up at that specialist (e.g., through referrals from their PCP).

4. **Fit.** Explore the type of business that the referring physician can and will shift to your facility. This can be as simple as getting additional MRIs from an orthopedic surgeon or understanding the PCP's need to send cardiac patients directly to a specialized type of cardiologist for a workup on their arrhythmia.

5. **Outcomes.** Encourage more referrals from physicians who represent the level of quality your organization wants to achieve. The organization will benefit from objectifying the facets of quality that come into play (e.g., length of stay, readmissions, infection rates, and peer assessments). This is relatively easy when a physician splits between your facility and others but becomes more difficult when they have not referred to your facility in the past. In that case, organizations must rely on word of

mouth and the traditional credentialing background tools. If you are in an academic medical center, part of the process must include evaluation of credentials. The other part of this is accepting all referrals and working with the referring physician to let them know when it is appropriate to make future referrals.

6. **Relationships.** Carefully consider who is encouraged to join or become more active in the ranks of the medical staff. The number-one challenge in this regard is the role of leadership in managing internal politics and relationships. The community hospital, with all private-practice physicians, is often forced to take a position that is counter to the desires of the existing specialists. There are times when it is absolutely the right thing to do to increase the number of specialists. Best-practice organizations are able to step back and clearly think through the impact. Generally, they also communicate with the current specialty group in a proactive way if they opt to encourage more business from another group. Another element of relationships is the prospective target's ability to get along with others. The bottom line is that if you are going to spend the resources to encourage new referrals, it makes sense to make sure they are good citizens within the medical staff. Watch for signs of trouble: past bad behavior in the operating room, jumping from practice to practice, or moving from facility to facility, for example. Again, this is much easier to assess if the physician is already sending you some referrals. Otherwise, use good judgment, and proceed with caution.

7. **Motivation.** Consider the need of referring physicians to grow their own business, too. There has to be some gain for them; otherwise, they are not going to be interested in changing their referral patterns. Some factors that motivate referring physicians include the following:

- Access to new insurance plans or the need to shore up the payer mix within the practice

- Prestige and recognition

- Technology and innovation

- A move for personal or business reasons

- New patients and more primary care referrals to grow their practice (for specialists)

- Specialists with better outcomes, clinical communication, and personal or social connections (for PCPs)

- Better support for PCPs, including hospitalist coverage, transport, or triage experts

One group that is often overlooked is physicians in your geographic market who are new to practice. Physicians in your service area—assuming that they are competent and will fit with your organization—who have been in practice for less than two years are the "right target," whether their practice is affiliated with you or not. Also, there may be new physicians in the market who joined groups that have not historically used your facility. It's a mistake to presume that they will follow the practice patterns of their existing practice. Although the initial tendency is to follow those patterns, often new physicians are interested in creating their own referral relationships. Let them know that you are available and what you have to offer. Clearly, there's more to targeting the right physician than just picking a few doctors from a list. The organizations that have done an exceptional job of growing their referrals have taken the time to decide objectively who to include in their targeted lists.

## Focus on your long-range vision and goals

Best-practice organizations maintain focus over time. When a program begins, there is a wonderful air of enthusiasm. The focal point of the program is a field-focused effort to enhance relationships and gain referrals. Although not everyone agrees—ever—about what to promote or who to promote it to, everyone shares the belief that the representative should be in the field meeting with physicians. Outcomes-focused programs often have key benchmarks to be achieved (e.g., a certain number of physician visits per week), making the program's path feel well established. With the key vulnerability typically including keeping field people in the field and creating a culture of referral readiness, the other enemy of focus happens over time: It is the lack of motivation to reexamine the plan and the approach.

         **A Marketer's Guide to Physician Relations**

Although the original targets and target list were painstakingly developed, subsequent lists are built by give-and-take, year after year. Those programs that have been able to maintain their focus commit to a fresh look at the data. Although there is tremendous value to long-term relationships, additions to and deletions from the list will be necessary. New physicians move in while others move to levels within the organization that demand the attention of leadership instead of the physician relations program. Markets change, and so do strategic priorities. Focus is about looking again at the reason for the program and then assessing which physicians to target and by whom, how the physician should be targeted, and when to meet the goal.

Beth Israel Deaconess Medical Center in Boston regularly reassesses its physician relations strategy. Elaine Monico, director of network development, says that Beth Israel looks at its strategy and approach about every six months. "From a market standpoint, how to achieve volume growth is really challenging in a market that is essentially flat," she says. "The last two or three years we have only seen in the range of 0.05% to 1% market growth. So we continuously have to look at what we offer and how we differentiate ourselves, given how formidable our competitors are, to achieve volume results."

The final enemy of focus is the temptation of incorporating too many good things into the program. There is a tendency to get very enthusiastic about the program and then add new elements to the program, including more things that can be done with and for doctors. Pretty soon, the consistency is replaced by a whole series of other, different, and special events. Sue Pietrafeso, director of outreach programs at Sunrise Health Systems in Las Vegas, calls this the magpie syndrome. You start out with the right idea but get distracted by shiny things. Focus eludes the magpie.

Take the time to formally assess your program every couple years. Look at the original goals of the program compared with the current goals. Have they changed? Look at the structure. Is it meeting the current needs? Do the representatives have the visibility and influence necessary to perform in their roles? Are they spending the right proportion of time in the field versus the office? Assess the strategic targets and the effect on referrals and volumes. Evaluate your internal communication plan, and see whether it is time to formalize it a bit. Best-practice facilities take the assessment seriously and do it right. Program focus requires that you take the time to learn what is in place to meet your goals, create a plan and process to meet the goals, and then build a message to attract others to the cause.

# Senior leadership involvement

## Build success from the top down

The pace and demands of executive teams at hospitals, health systems, and large physician practices have grown exponentially in recent years. Every day brings new challenges, not only in physician relations but also in areas such as technology, employee and payer relations, allocation of resources, the physical plant, and myriad others. In addition, the competitive environment is just that—competitive. (Actually, in some markets, the better term might be cutthroat.) With all the mission-critical issues that demand their attention, why should senior leaders make the physician relations program a top priority? Because the program will never be truly successful unless senior leaders—including the CEO, other members of the C-suite, and physician leaders—are actively involved.

Physicians are bright people. They'll figure out very quickly whether the physician relations program has the power, influence, and commitment of the senior leaders behind it. Many of us who have grown up in marketing and business development have actively participated in successful programs that were *willed* from the ground up. Physician relations, however, is not one of those programs. In best-practice organizations, support from the program comes from the top down. Consider the following:

- Physicians form opinions about a healthcare organization based on its leaders. No matter what lower-level employees do or say, it is the leaders who create the impression.

- Physicians will quickly assess whether your message is aligned with your actions. They'll lose trust in the relationship if they think leaders are only paying lip service to it.

- Physicians compare institutions. Their intrinsic nature is to diagnose almost every situation—and it's easier for them to rule out your organization than it is to change their habits and rule you in. The prospective physician is rarely interested in testing you or taking a trial run at referring their patients to your care. If they are going to shift business, they will move through their methodical deductive process of determining why they should *not* refer patients to your organization. A key factor in their decision is whether senior leaders are aware and involved in the desire to have them shift their business and whether that desire is based on all the right reasons, for both the physician and the organization.

   **A Marketer's Guide to Physician Relations**

Many leaders say they are totally supportive of the physician relations effort. And I take them at their word. But in best-practice organizations, leaders don't just say they support the program: They take actionable efforts to support it. Senior leaders who are involved in the physician relations program have a positive impact on sales effectiveness. To grow the relationship with a referring physician, the physician relations representative must have the right level of knowledge and the ability to get things done. The salesperson must be confident that if he or she says someone from the organization will address the physician's concern, then that person will respond in a timely manner. Only senior leaders have the clout to make that happen.

The salesperson also needs pertinent details about happenings within the organization that he or she can pass on to the physician—the kind of information that comes from the top. Too often, representatives waste valuable time trying to create an aura of effectiveness and value without really having the internal power to make things happen.

### *Leaders help open doors*

There was a time when physicians welcomed a visit from the hospital representative, who would catch them up on what was new at the hospital. These days, practices are absolutely inundated with representatives pitching pharmaceuticals, medical equipment, alternative-treatment programs, and a host of hospitals. Most people hate being sold to. As a result, more and more practices are saying no to sales visits.

To be effective today, the representative must take a different approach to stand apart from other sales representatives. He or she must provide a distinct level of information and expertise, create a position of value within the mind of the physician, and consistently deliver on the promises that he or she makes. This is clearly not the friendly little "tell and sell" or "find and fix" representative of the past.

To effectively build a relationship, the physician relations representative must get quality time with the physician. And that's where active support from leadership can give the representative a distinct advantage. If I told you I was coming to visit your hospital today, what would you do? If your schedule happened to be light that day, you might try to make time to talk to me. But on a busy day? I'd probably be out of luck, right? But what if I were to tell you that the governor of your state asked me to stop in and connect with you? You'd likely be more willing to lend me an ear, regardless of your political persuasion.

Most people like to know that key decision makers, especially those who have an impact on their lives, value their opinions. If the representative comes to the physician's office armed with a message from the leadership of his or her organization and prepared to have a quality, two-way conversation, the physician will feel more positive about the experience. He or she will feel that the organization values his or her opinions. That's what makes the physician representative's face-to-face meeting stand apart from the typical sales meeting with someone who is pushing a product.

**A Marketer's Guide to Physician Relations**

Best-practice organizations recognize that the physician relations program works only if the representative can connect with the physician. To help accomplish that goal, they make it clear to referring physicians that the representative is an extension of the organization's leaders, that he or she is their presence in the field. Leaders at best-practice organizations are comfortable allowing the representative to use their position and name recognition to open doors and appointment books. They are at ease with the representative as an extension of their efforts because they are confident that the representative will act well on their behalf.

Getting in the door is only half the battle, however. There is another element of success that also relies heavily on the right level of leadership support. Physician relations representatives at best-practice organizations provide enough depth during the field visit to allow for a professional exchange. The goal is that, once the representative has made it though the physician's door one or two times, he or she will be welcomed back on a regular basis.

To do this, the representative must engage in dialogue (and not merely try to sell to the physician) and use his or her knowledge and communication skills to create the opportunity for more referrals. At best-practice organizations, the representative is a high-level professional who is able to articulate the nuances that differentiate the organization and its services. He or she must ask quality questions and clearly understand the physician's needs. And he or she must be able to disclose appropriate details about the strategic direction when needed.

That is where the connection and commitment of senior leaders come into play. The physician's primary concern is doing what is best for his or her patients. That's what physicians do. If we are trying to change their beliefs about what facility offers the best care, we must make a compelling case. This is not accomplished with fast talk; it is accomplished with *credible* talk. This level of knowledge surely requires top-notch talent, but it also means that the representative is privy to the right depth and breadth of knowledge from the organization's leadership and that he or she knows how and when to use it. It is the right kind of information at the right level, so the physician really believes that the representative is an extension of the organization's leadership.

Innate to this level of positioning is a two-fold obligation: The representative must be of the appropriate professional level to deserve the information and to manage it well, and the leadership must be willing to step forward, provide the detail, and give the representative a chance to turn the information into a successful relationship with the physician.

## Attributes of involved leaders

There are several leadership qualities that demonstrate involvement. CEOs at best-practice organizations share the following characteristics:

- They ensure buy-in from members of the leadership team

- They frequently articulate the strategic goals and priorities for physician relations

- They show concern for physicians' issues, even though they are different from their own

- They give representatives information that is relevant for communication and for positioning the organization

- They accompany the representative on field visits from time to time

- They show visible support for strategically selected service lines that are responsive to the physician relations team

- They do not rely only on the carrot but are willing to use the stick if needed

- They give the person who has oversight for the physician relations program enough autonomy to innovate

- They hold the field staff accountable for results but also provide them with a working system that can deliver minimum expectations consistently

### *The best leaders build internal support*

Once the stage is set with good leadership support for efforts in the field, the next step is to employ foundational tools that support the physician-relations effort with those inside the facility. Some of these practices will vary depending on the organization, while others are important for all organizations. Senior leaders who are actively engaged in this process will tell you that they have had a bit of trial and error. They will also tell you that they have had some hugely successful results with this process.

Beth Israel Deaconess Medical Center in Boston needed to grow its surgical volume to achieve its necessary financial benchmarks, so the organization set out on a multipronged effort that included both internal and external efforts. The first step was to recruit the needed surgical talent that would distinguish the medical center from the other tertiary facilities in Boston. Coupled with that effort, the CEO charged the chief of surgery with redesigning the surgical compensation system so that the surgeons would be rewarded personally for gains in surgical volume. Once those pieces were in place, the physician relations and marketing teams were charged with building awareness for the surgical services and increasing the surgical referral volume from community-based physicians.

The key element that makes this a best practice is laying the foundation with the clinical services offerings and surgeon incentives so that the there would be the right synergy in place to make the outreach efforts effective. CEOs at best-practice organizations actively spread the message about their physician relations programs to all stakeholders, and especially to other members of the internal leadership team.

Some CEOs will tell you that this is much more difficult than they thought it would be. One CEO I know had successfully employed a similar sales program at a previous facility with great success. At a senior leadership meeting, he

**A Marketer's Guide to Physician Relations**

announced that we would be consulting with the team to develop a new physician relations/sales initiative. He talked enthusiastically about his past success and then asked us to share our process with the team. We discussed the role of each member of the leadership team. All listened. The CEO asked for questions, there were none, and the meeting came to an end. There were many fits and starts over the next four months, with battles over internal data, challenges in completing the hiring process, and angst about the reporting roles and goals. When we returned for the next meeting with leadership, it was clear to the CEO and to us that the other senior executives did not believe in the program and were not actively supporting it. Despite what their boss had said, some were sure it was a flash-in-the-pan idea that was not worthy of the effort. A couple of them felt the program was intruding on their own turf. They considered themselves the "owners" of the doctor relationships.

Sometimes internal resistance is not this blatant. But members of the senior team can fail to support the physician relations program for a variety of reasons. If the CEO is able to recognize and deal with this early on, the road to success will be much smoother.

Steps to success include holding frequent meetings to discuss the need for the program and the CEO's expectations. The internal communication plan (discussed in Chapter 1) will also help, as will making others in the leadership ranks responsible for the program's success. Those who do it well have recognized early on that this is not a one-department program. The physician relations program will be more successful—and be successful sooner—when it has organizationwide involvement and support.

### *The best leaders manage the message*

With the internal stakeholders on board, consider methods to create consistent messages regarding special areas of interest for physicians. Message management is a really big deal these days, in part because of the pace, the variety of communication tools, and the unpredictable nature of the hospital work flow. When members of the leadership team have the chance to connect with the medical staff, it's important to have quality messages to share with them. Leaders should be able to share proactive comments, inform the medical staff about events and topics of interest, or simply recognize them for their contributions to the organization.

Some leaders use modern tools to help manage the messages. Blogs and other communication vehicles give the CEO a consistent forum to deliver the organization's message to both internal and external audiences.

The other category worthy of prepared communication is the crafting of messages around hot topics. There are times when every organization must make unpopular decisions. This could be anything from a change in nursing leadership within a unit to plans for a joint venture with one of three area cardiology groups for a freestanding catheterization laboratory. Often those who support the decision have a clear understanding of the message and what should and should not be communicated. Others, even within the leadership team, may not. When a physician catches a leader at a volunteer function and asks about goings-on at the hospital, there is tremendous value in being able to provide the same answer as every other leader regardless of whether he or she is directly involved in the project. The same goes for the physician relations

**A Marketer's Guide to Physician Relations**

representative. In fact, it's even more important for the representative to have the right message ready, since the physician will usually feel safe probing for details with the representative. When there are hot issues, best-practice organizations prepare the messages so everyone is on the same page and gives a consistent answer.

## *The best leaders articulate the strategic goals*

New programs are usually developed with an objective approach and linked closely to the organization's strategic plan. The long-term ability to link the day-to-day efforts with the global needs of the organization necessarily falls to the organization's leaders. Those who do it well are determined and consistent in keeping the plan on course.

So why is that so hard? Because when you ask someone to work closely with the medical staff, you will unearth a multitude of other opportunities. Beyond the challenges with focus that we described in Chapter 1, many departments and services are eager to grow but may not be part of the strategic plan. The organization benefits if the leadership takes a stand on this and provides the big-picture thinking and rationale for the suggested process. The physician relations team is generally not in a position to make this decision. Midlevel managers do not feel comfortable telling service-line leaders that their program may not be the right one to position proactively. Setting priorities is the mechanism for this. Forward-thinking leadership teams take the time to reexamine and communicate priorities on a yearly basis. This is a great time for senior leaders to say that they have asked the physician relations team to target this year's growth effort on (for example) orthopedics, neurosurgery, and outpatient imaging. This sets the stage for providing the physician relations team with expected outcomes.

At CHRISTUS Schumpert Health System in Shreveport, LA, CEO Joe Paine and Lori Marshall, manager of physician relations, business, and industry, have developed a process that works well for them. For each service line (e.g., oncology), they ask several questions. Is it profitable? Is it an industry leader? Is it a gateway to other service lines? Is it cutting edge and/or does it help physician satisfaction? "Then we select which services lines are 'fit' for physician relations support," says Marshall. "There's only three of us, so we can't do everything and do it well."

### The best leaders apply filters

Leaders from best-practice organizations—those who have continued to grow their physician relations programs either in influence or in size—have learned to value the unique external perspective that the physician relations team brings to the table. This filter allows leaders to see the organization from the outside. The best leaders rely on the physician relations team to share this perspective. It might not always cause them to change their opinions, but this kind of insight only helps the relationship.

### The best leaders see both sides

Leaders at best-practice organizations take their role in creating the right environment for success seriously. They work to set an example by exemplifying behaviors that demonstrate interest in the physicians and their needs. They recognize that the physician practice is the entry point for success.

All leaders readily acknowledge this, yet it is easy to get caught up in hospital challenges and forget that the physician has his or her own challenges. Both share the challenge of meeting patient needs and negotiating with managed care, but when it comes to the daily issues of practice, most resemble a small business, compared with the big-business entity of a hospital. Strong leadership teams diligently work to evaluate both sides of the story: to keep abreast of market intelligence and to understand changes in the practice and lifestyle needs of their medical staff. Most leaders understand this. But best-practice leaders show the physicians upon whom they rely for additional growth that they are empathetic to the realities of today's practitioner.

At Columbus (OH) Children's Hospital, Donna Teach, vice president (VP) of market development and promotion, employs a medical-level champion to help the organization achieve this best practice. The champion is responsible for issue resolution and setting service standards. And although those standards have been established, the champion also is sensitive to the specific requests from referring physicians who might need something different based on the acuity of a referral.

### The best leaders make field visits

In best-practice organizations, the CEO gets involved in the right field efforts. He or she might be there to listen and learn, to manage a specific issue, or to get acquainted with a physician. The representative should know when a CEO's visit would add value. I would encourage the CEO to use this time to learn about the physician's practice and to learn more about how the representative functions. It is a wonderful, visible sign of support.

Consider meeting with key specialists but also with internists, pediatricians, and family physicians. Because hospitalist use is so prevalent, there is less connection between hospitals and primary care physicians (PCP). A meeting with the hospital CEO or a top member of the leadership team can go a long way in creating an identity for the organization in the mind of the PCP. Although there are times during the visit when the leader should take over the conversation, it's okay for the leader to engage but allow the representative to have an active role in leading the dialogue.

### The best leaders use the carrot and the stick

Within the relationship strategy, there is ample opportunity to get good mileage from a carrot approach—extolling and rewarding the behavior you desire. This, of course, works marvelously well for encouraging referral growth. There are also some great opportunities to highlight the efforts of service leaders who embrace the relationship sales efforts. It is great to do this one-on-one, but if you want other service line leaders to emulate the behavior, it's more effective to give praise in front of the group. Here are some examples of the type of activities that are ripe for recognition:

- Operational leaders who assist with on-site presentations or meetings with the targeted physician

- Service line leaders who work hard to create a solid solution when physicians complain

**A Marketer's Guide to Physician Relations**

- Departments/services that provide outcome data to position and differentiate their area above the competitor

- Clinical areas that are gracious to new physicians and go the extra mile to make them feel welcome

- Services—especially outpatient and clinic appointments—that proactively explore systems of access from the vantage point of internal needs and the view of the customer/referring practice

Praise from the leadership team goes miles in creating the right type of collaboration. But don't rely on the carrot only; if you need the stick, use it. Disciplinary action can help gain consistency and support for the program. Consider discipline in circumstances such as the following:

- The operations team members do not meet service standards or follow through on requests from physicians that are relayed by the physician representatives

- Department leaders and staff aren't welcoming to new physicians

- Members of the leadership team see the gathering of physician issues as an opportunity to get some "dirt" or use information to hurt a colleague purposefully

## Autonomy and innovation

There is no question that physicians are vital to the success of most healthcare organizations today. It is no wonder that members of the leadership team feel a level of vulnerability in turning over relationship building. The challenge is balancing involvement versus control.

In Chapter 1, we talked about the challenge that occurs when a leader believes that his or her approach to building internal relationships is the right approach to replicate in the field. The suggestions are all very well intended but may not always enhance the approach. In fact, sometimes they are detrimental. If you have hired a representative who is a relationship expert, then it's wise to let the representative use his or her style and approach to create the right relationship sales environment. Here are some ways that best-practice leaders encourage autonomy in the physician relations representative:

- When they offer suggestions, they make it clear that they are options— not expectations.

- They strive to create a vision of what they hope for as a part of the new relationship. They focus on this vision, not on the tactical path to get there, to allow the representative to decide how best to accomplish the task.

- They recognize that most salespeople will occasionally go a bit too far, promising something that operations must struggle to deliver, for

**A Marketer's Guide to Physician Relations**

example. They let the representative know that this is not acceptable but do not draw the line on what the representative can say or how he or she should say it. Remember, we value sales professionals because, to them, no never really means no—even if that sometimes makes them difficult to manage.

- They give the representative reasonable boundaries by setting a few (three or four) very clear ground rules. For example, they might ask representatives not to share certain information or to have a stock response to a certain question.

- They create opportunities to learn from the representatives and others about what helps them make connections in the field.

- They give the person who has oversight enough autonomy to innovate. With all the interest in connecting with the physician, there is an excellent opportunity to create new, different approaches, which might include a unique way to get the physician's attention, a new technique to make connections among specialists, or a new idea about how to get PCPs more engaged. New ideas can create positive energy for the team.

- They do not encourage innovation at the expense of the program's overall goal, however. New ideas must not distract from the field effort, must be shown to have measurable impact within a set trial period, and must have no (or limited) downside. In addition, the cost of the plan or idea must be weighed against the benefit to the physician.

# Harnessing market intelligence

In best-practice organizations, leaders benefit from the wealth of field intelligence gleaned by the representative. In the course of a day, representatives are exposed to several physicians and others in the physicians' offices. They also come in contact with other representatives and with community stakeholders.

Business opportunities and partnerships and relationships with physicians are constantly changing in today's climate. The earlier the leaders can get reliable information, the better. With ears wide open, physician relations representatives will naturally hear conversations on a wide range of topics, including competitive information, the health of the physician's business, and market perceptions. The internal approach is to encourage the physician relations staff to listen for and provide details about these topics. This must be thought out ahead of time and done with the right intentions, however— one would never want a practice to think that the representative is just there to gather intelligence, and the representatives' first priority is to create relationships and grow referrals.

To find this balance, explain when and how the representative should gather this kind of information and give them some background for context. For example, if the representative is going to visit Dr. Smith and the leadership has been speaking with him about purchasing his practice, the representative should know this. Ask the representative to check for outward signs of change in the practice. If the physician mentions the purchase, tell the representative to get details about the time frame or any barriers that are slowing the process.

     **A Marketer's Guide to Physician Relations**

Although physicians will often share information of this nature, it is important for the representative to know how to ask the right questions to clearly understand if it is just "talk" or if it is reality. The role of the representative is to discern the background, timelines, emotions, and authenticity when statements are made within the categories of market intelligence. In addition, there are times when the representative should ask the physician whether the details the physician is sharing can be communicated within the organization.

Internal leaders need to respect the nature of the representative's relationship with the referring physician and realize that there are times when the physician is speaking in confidence. This is rare, however, because generally the physician wants leadership to know what he or she is thinking; it is the reason the physician tells the representative. Physician relations representatives at best-practice organizations look for information in several different categories:

**Information about competitors:**
- Facility building and expansion plans

- New partners

- New partnerships and affiliations

- Trouble, departures, and/or changes in leadership—especially within departments

- Field presence

## Information about practices:

- Changes within the practice partners—recruitment, retirement, switching to part-time status

- Challenges with the business side of medicine—malpractice, business management

- Restructuring within the practice

- Issues with partners, including a physician who wants to leave

## Information about market perceptions:

- Buzz and opinions, especially following media coverage of a health-related event

- Concerns about the viability of organizations or departments, especially after the departure of a high-profile leader or physician

- Changing opinions about the market leader or quality

- Response to or interest in recent marketing promotions

Use intelligence from representatives to alert you to changes in momentum. Those organizations that are working to gain favorable momentum among the community or the medical staff will have more buzz in the marketplace. CHRISTUS Schumpert's Paine looks at the physician relations effort as an

**A Marketer's Guide to Physician Relations**

opportunity to acquire information that goes beyond a straight sales effort. Representatives gather intelligence on "recruitment, retention, competitor actions, and other things like that," he says. "Actually, our entire recruitment agenda bounced off the sales group."

Equally important is knowing what to do with the intelligence once gathered. When programs are young, there is a great deal of adulation over intelligence details. Truth be told, the tendency is likely to have too many involved and to react with too much intensity. However, as programs mature, they often fall into a solid pattern of managing intelligence. Sometimes, if the information is about medical staff relations, the information is shared personally with the chief medical officer. Depending on the level of information, the VP who has oversight may accompany the representative to share the knowledge with the CEO. Routine intelligence can be included in the monthly report.

There is one last nuance that likely goes without saying, but it is about the nimbleness of the best leaders to use what is learned in a positive and proactive way. Some of the information that is learned will feel personal, so the tendency is to defend or defuse the credibility of the intelligence.

Those who do it well work hard to step back and look at the information from the point of view of the referring physician and then find a middle ground. They find a way to respond to the representative in a way that thanks the representative for sharing. They share details about their response (or lack of response) with the representative so that he or she can learn from it.

In so doing, they further hone the skills of the representatives; they learn to be shrewder in gathering details, and the leaders again are the beneficiaries. Those who are the best-practice leaders work to close the loop with the representatives who bring market intelligence forward.

In summary, senior leadership's involvement in physician relations is more than a nice addition. Every program benefits from this, whether it is to get things started, to gain credibility, or to keep the program focused and on track. When the senior leadership team is actively involved, there is better attention to the details of responsiveness. The outcome is that relationships are valued and managed well. It commits the organization to a position that states each physician's experience with us is important, each time.

# 3

 # Capable staff

## Hire your way to a winning program

No physician relations program can be successful without the right people to staff it. Some organizations take a scientific approach to hiring, and almost all conduct multiple interviews to help find the best talent for the job. But here's the tricky thing: Individuals who are good at selling are naturally going to be good at selling themselves during the interview. Best-practice organizations work hard to manage this.

Although critical to success, hiring capable staff is obviously about more than just finding good people. Best-practice organizations not only take painstaking effort to find the right people but also recognize their obligation to help them to succeed in the role. Best-practice organizations use solid tools and techniques to orient, integrate, motivate, and guide sales staff. Some employ extensive performance management tools, some use incentive-based compensation, and others have tight reporting and senior leadership accountability as a part of their approach. All the best-practice programs have solid systems in place for finding, training, motivating, and rewarding the right talent for the role.

Consider these three important benefits of hiring the right person for the role:

- **Results.** Talented salespeople have the ability to get quality time with the desired group of physicians and provide focused messages that result in increased referrals. They are not just putting in the effort but being strategic about how they sell to get referrals and results more quickly.

- **Physician acceptance.** The right representative will be someone whom the physician will welcome into his or her practice. Physicians want someone they can trust, who will get them solid information, and who is not trying to sell them something. They also value someone who understands their world—the challenges of practice, the clinical expectations of their specialty, the needs of their patients, and the business challenges they face—someone, in short, who can empathize with them.

- **Internal fit.** The right person will also bring internal credibility to the program. It is important to have someone who can earn the respect of the key internal stakeholders and the confidence of leaders. This, in turn, results in better-quality internal interactions around the physicians. Sometimes a representative has the skill to create external relationships but just can't seem to get the internal team to support his or her efforts. Although this internal trust and respect can be earned in the long run, it is so much easier and more effective to hire someone who has the internal support right from the beginning.

## How to find the right person for the job

When hiring within healthcare, we often work with our HR departments to evaluate the right "fit" for jobs. That includes determining who is ideal for the job or, alternatively, the person who is acceptable for the position. For many healthcare jobs, we can hire people who are acceptable or adequate. We know that if they are willing, we can train them. But this doesn't always work for the physician relations program. When it comes to hiring someone for this position, it is critical that the candidate have the ability to sell. Most facilities do not have the expertise to teach new hires sales techniques. Almost without exception, this means that the organization must hire someone who already has sales ability. The key word is ability—meaning the person has an aptitude for selling.

> *I don't know how much of it is nature versus nurture. You can learn how to sell, but if it's hardwired in your DNA, it just makes it so much easier.*

— Roger Smith, vice president (VP) of HR, *HCA Continental Division*

The need to find, measure, and evaluate sales ability is complicated by the fact that the HR team may not have the expertise to evaluate sales aptitude. To manage this challenge, some facilities give the task to someone on the HR staff who has recruited for sales in previous positions.

"What worked for me is that I got personally involved in the project," says Roger Smith, VP of HR at HCA Continental Division in Denver, who was charged with hiring a new VP of sales. "I was connected at the hip with the CEO, who was assigned to implement the project, so I was personally vested in making sure it was a success."

Best-practice organizations, including HCA Continental, supplement their internal efforts with external resources, such as an external recruiter, screener, or consultant who specializes in conducting sales interviews. They use every resource available to find the right talent.

### External resources

Some organizations rely on outside resources to find and screen talent because the task is outside their normal scope of expertise. There are recruiters who have expertise in this area, but you will want to carefully screen them to find the right firm for the level of expertise you desire.

"Finding a healthcare-exclusive recruiter may not be as critical for this type of assignment," says Mike Frommelt, principal and cofounder of KeyStone Search, a recruitment firm in Minneapolis. It's more important to find a search firm that can identify the right talent based on competencies, he adds. In other words, the firm must be able to look at candidates' skills, background, work habits, and values and determine whether a he or she would be right for the physician relations position. Some search firms are simply "background brokers," maintaining a large database of potential candidates and shifting them around according to need. Given that physician relations is a relatively new and emerging field, it is important that the recruiter can go deeper than just filling a slot—the recruiter must be able to evaluate the candidate's possibility for success in the new role based on successes in other, disparate arenas. The firm must be able to evaluate talent at a deeper level and to assess your organization's culture, direction, and strategic vision and incorporate that information into the search for the ideal candidate.

In addition to recruitment firms, there are national companies that profile the ideal attributes needed for a candidate to succeed in a role and then test the top candidates to gauge their aptitude for the job. Smith got good results with an assessment tool. "We're looking for someone who is a natural-born seller, someone who is hardwired for sales. Although these tools aren't 100% reliable, we are better off having used it than not at the end of the day. We can with more confidence make a hire and say we have four data points that tell me this is the right candidate for the position—the interview, references, résumé, and the assessment tool." The tool helped Smith measure cognitive strength (the ability to analyze numbers and think in words), behavior (persistence, energy level, and sociability), and motivation (the kinds of things a person likes to do).

There are several other methods to consider when using outside sources to recruit physician relations representatives. One option is to hire an expert to conduct a telephone interview. If the HR team is not accustomed to screening for selling skills, you may opt to use an outside expert to conduct a telephone interview with the top candidates to evaluate their sales ability and whether they're fit for the role. Although the external consultant won't be able to assess whether a candidate is a good fit with your internal culture, the consultant can evaluate the candidate's aptitude for developing relationship sales opportunities with physicians. Another option is to create an internal selection process. Many facilities need no outside support; they successfully develop internal tools to identify and screen the right candidates for the role. Whether you do it on your own or you get a little help, it is important to recognize the attributes that are important.

## Attributes of the right person

The right person is someone who positions the organization and its leadership in a favorable way to the physicians. He or she can connect—listening, communicating, and using education and relationship skills—to encourage new referrals. Best-practice organizations hire the kind of person whom physicians see as an excellent resource, someone they can trust to handle details and get them the help they need. There are several attributes needed for the role.

### Knowledge
Those who are most effective can quickly assimilate medical knowledge and have strong oral and written communication skills. Good grammar and

**A Marketer's Guide to Physician Relations**

enunciation are little things that can become big things when working to gain credibility. The right candidate will understand the deductive reasoning process and use strong analogies to create interest and connections. The right candidate is quick to acknowledge when he or she doesn't have the answer and will work to find the right person to provide accurate details.

Doctors often turn to trusted advisors for other matters, such as insurance, banking, or nonpractice business. There is tremendous value in creating that level of rapport, and it starts with the right cognition. These individuals leverage their knowledge and then use some of the other attributes listed below to position integrity in the relationship. Knowledge is also about having the right background and expertise for the service lines and healthcare entities that they are hoping to grow. If the candidate has a healthcare background, he or she likely comes out ahead on pure product knowledge. If they do not come from this background, it can be learned with the right drive and aptitude for learning.

When you are interviewing, pay attention to how quickly the candidate responds and the depth of the response. Try asking some multipronged questions, and test how the candidate works through the answers. For example, ask the candidate how he or she would go about the process of learning about your organization and the services.

## Persistence

This job demands more than a little tenacity and persistence to make the difference. Having said that, we are not looking for an aggressive person who won't take no for an answer. Although everyone wants more business, for the physician relations representative, there is much more to be gained than a short-term yes from the physician. And if that yes occurs simply because the physician felt bullied into it, he or she might not follow through. With long-term sales, the key is to build a relationship that creates business on the physician's terms for all the right reasons.

> "This job is not for the weak of heart. They have to be bold—not necessarily pushy, but bold."
>
> — Mike Riley, VP of sales, *HCA Continental Division*

The ideal candidate finds innovative ways to engage the prospective physician in dialogue and increase the physician's interest in the services provided. Persistence takes the form of regular meetings on topics of interest for the referring physician. It is about looking for nuances in approach and style. Best-practice organizations look for the kind of personality type that experiences joyful glee when he or she takes business away from a competitor. To screen for this, ask the candidate to describe a time when he or she beat out a competitor. Look for a candidate who lights up at the chance to tell the story, who talks about out-thinking and outpositioning the competitor, and who wins with finesse.

### Work style

Work style includes work ethic, work volume, and work methods. Each has its own characteristics, and because a strong relationship salesperson is likely "selling you" in the interview, it's important to determine ahead of time how you value and judge this attribute. We would never hire someone who admits in an interview to doing the least amount of work possible to get a paycheck,

   **A Marketer's Guide to Physician Relations**

but this is the motivation for some employees. And although it is hard to manage these folks when they are working in-house in your department, the challenge increases tenfold when they are working in the field.

When interviewing for this role, ask candidates how they would create their weekly implementation plans. Ask them to share when they anticipate having appointments with physicians, and see whether they assume the physician will work around their schedule or if they see themselves working around the needs of the referring physician. Are they looking for a structured 9 a.m. to 5 p.m. position? If you get that impression, then push further through scenarios to determine whether they can and will work as you need them to.

Work methods are very much about individual style and how one approaches the job. Those who do well have the discipline to make the appointments and the curiosity and drive to be spontaneous in their approach to the role. In real life, that plays out in their ability to have not only the requisite 12 scheduled appointments every week but also the desire to schedule one more when they see the opportunity.

> *We need to assess the extent to which salespeople are normally independent. Working with physicians, we need people who welcome support and appreciate the need for procedure but don't depend on it. I want both high independence and collaboration.*
>
> — Roger Smith, VP of human resources, *HCA Continental Division*

## Commitment

The key to commitment is to find someone who, once trained and developed, will stay with you. It's tough, especially in today's environment where, with so many new programs starting, there is a tendency to poach existing talent from other facilities. Again, this is not unique to physician relations—every department wants to minimize turnover. However, once deep and trusting relationships are forged, changes in staff cost time, erode trust, and slow referral momentum. Be alert to indications that the candidate sees the job as a stepping stone. For example, if the interviewee asks about the path for advancement in this role, take the opportunity to ask more about the interviewee's long-term aspirations and the path and timeline that the interviewee has set for himself or herself.

## Ability to listen

I often say we are hired for sales roles because we are great talkers. Yet the most important quality of sales is being a good listener. It is critically important that the physician relations representative knows how to ask good questions and then has the ability to listen well and comprehend the reply. When listening is well done, the reply often leads to a higher level of dialogue and clearly provides indications about the physician's needs. Good listeners will pick up on statements you make during the interview process. They use phrases such as "Tell me more about that." They come to the interview prepared with first-rate questions. When you ask good listeners a question during an interview, they will answer it succinctly and then shift the focus back to you.

## *Likability*

It is very important that you find the candidate engaging, warm, and genuinely likable right off the bat. Although likability is a hard attribute to quantify, physicians should instantly feel compelled to converse with the representative. An element of the likability quotient is sincerity. The person must be genuine and have strong people skills. I once hired a person who had all the right attributes on paper, but I did not really connect with him on a personal level. It was a disaster—not because it was all him and not me, but because no one in the practices cared much about his background. They cared about their own needs, and he simply could not ingratiate himself to create a relationship. This attribute is easy to gauge in an interview: Do you connect with the person or not? In addition to being likable, the representative must genuinely enjoy spending time with physicians. The representative doesn't have to be in awe of them, but it does not work if the representative sees physicians as egotistical pains to work with. To do this job, the representative has to appreciate physicians and the work they do.

## *Intuition and flexibility*

Intuition is an attribute that I had personally overlooked until I spent some time with someone who did not possess it. Intuition is that ability to "read" the physician and his or her practice; it's knowing when the physician is interested and relating to you or when the physician is bored or too busy to take the time to have a meaningful conversation. Personally, I would not hire anyone who did not have strong intuitive skills and the ability to quickly assess other people and the environment. The ability to think along with the prospective physician and to read his or her body language and to intuit his or her interests is an important differentiator. To test this, toward the end of the interview, glance at your watch when the candidate responds to a question. It's a red flag if the candidate continues to talk.

Flexibility goes with intuition because it plays out as an extension of the same. If the physician relations representative intuits that the physician is too busy or too preoccupied to meet, he or she must be flexible. When you interview, you can get a sense of the candidate's flexibility when you are trying to set up interviews or calls. If the candidate works to accommodate you, he or she probably understands the value of flexibility when you are working to get something you want.

## Self-esteem

Self-esteem may seem a bit pop psychology, but it's definitely something to consider and evaluate in a physician relations candidate. Besides the fact that people with high self-esteem tend to be more capable of handling rejection, even more importantly, they do not tend to make excuses or deflect blame. Nothing will kill a program faster than someone who makes excuses or looks to blame others or the rest of the organization when things don't go his or her way.

People with high self-esteem are confident and comfortable in their own skin, not arrogant or cocky. Arrogance is often a sign of low self-esteem—a person who is overly worried about how they appear to others. This is absolutely critical, as people who are arrogant will tend to be combative, and those who

**A Marketer's Guide to Physician Relations**

are overly self-deprecating or humble to a fault will have a difficult time building productive relationships with physicians and team members.

The best candidates are right in the middle, confident in their abilities but humble in their approach. "We have come to realize that excuse-makers can poison an organization wherever they reside," says Mike Frommelt from KeyStone Search. To evaluate self-esteem, ask the candidate to describe a project in which he or she was involved that failed. Ask what he or she would do differently. Candidates who cannot give an example of a failure are probably not being honest. Be wary of those who deflect blame. Look for those who talk honestly about a failure and who describe what they learned from the experience.

### Understanding what makes healthcare organizations tick

Hospitals differ from other businesses in that they are driven by operations. Although this is changing in light of new competition, the focus and attention are still on operations—not on sales and marketing—to grow business.

When people join a physician relations program and are charged with creating new referrals, they assume that everyone in the organization will be pleased and that there will be a concerted effort to be responsive to the needs of the physicians whom we want to join the ranks. In reality, that is not exactly true. I am not certain whether it is the complexity of the internal decision-making process or the challenges with changing old habits, but in most hospitals, the sales process is not embraced. For those who come from sales-driven organizations, this can be challenging and frustrating.

In my opinion, this attribute is not make-or-break, but it is important to be aware of so you can orient accordingly. If you don't and the person becomes frustrated with his or her lack of ability to have an impact on the internal organization, you risk losing this person. As you interview candidates, ask questions about what they would do and what they would expect others to do when a new physician admits a patient.

### Clinical background (maybe)

When I am asked about the right person, one of the first questions is often, "Should they have a clinical background or not?" The answer is that it depends on the individual and his or her other capabilities. It also depends on the type of service that you are working to grow and the maturity of other physician relations efforts in your market.

Over time, my opinion about this has changed a bit. I continue to believe that the most important attribute is the ability to develop the right relationships and gain commitment—in other words, good selling skills. However, I have come to believe that the candidate must also have the right level of clinical knowledge. Although it can be taught, it cannot be gained through osmosis from the healthcare culture. If your organization opts to hire a nonclinical person who has excellent sales skills, then you must give them a real education.

Some organizations I've worked with have been disappointed when their programs did not grow as much as they would have liked. When I assess their programs, I sometimes find that the sales staff does not have the tools to grow the communication to a deeper level. They are great at asking opening

© 2007 HCPRO, INC.    **A Marketer's Guide to Physician Relations**

questions and getting physician-to-physician meetings set up, but over time, they fail to create a more robust platform for knowledge because their clinical knowledge lacks the right depth. The bottom line is that if you hire a great salesperson, you must give them a robust orientation and ongoing clinical updates to expand his or her breadth of knowledge.

Empathy is an attribute that, although certainly not unique to nurses, is characteristic of many. This is a wonderful characteristic for relationship sales. Empathetic people naturally work to understand the needs of the other person, and they work hard to listen and learn. Also, clinical staffs certainly understand the scientific process, which relates to planning and decision-making. These qualities all help with connecting, but, of course, that is only part of successful growth.

So, if clinicians and caregivers have all these good qualities, why invest time training a nonclinical person? Why not just hire a nurse in the first place? Believe me when I say that an outstanding nurse can be a failure as a physician relations representative.

Many nurses went into the profession because they are wonderful problem solvers. They enjoy the caregiving process because they are able to take what is wrong and make it better. Although these attributes serve them well for patient care, and they work well for retention of existing referrals, they are not well suited for an individual charged with growth. The reason is that growth requires the physician relations representative to keep pressing forward with his or her targeted groups to share the messages and stay focused on growth.

Because clinical staff are often excellent problem solvers, they don't like to turn over the issues to others to solve. Rather, they like to actively work alongside the internal team to find a solution. But this is not the job of the field-focused physician representative.

To test how comfortable the candidate is with letting others fix problems, ask about an especially rewarding experience and evaluate the story that he or she shares. Was it about a problem that he or she resolved? If so, did the story focus on the process or the result? Listen for a story about a successful relationship that resulted in a gain for the candidate's place of employment.

You want to hire the candidate who doesn't want to fix everything that is broken and has the ability to continue in the role even if the deliverable is not perfect. He or she must also be comfortable asking the physician for some form of commitment. The role of the physician relations representative is to continue to move the relationship forward. When done well, there is an expected outcome for each visit as the representative creates a climate for ultimately gaining the referral opportunity. Some of the best nurses are conflict avoiders (i.e., consensus builders). They may not advance the relationship as quickly or with as clear a path as someone who has a traditional sales aptitude. Again, good training can help overcome this.

Some nurses want to get out of the profession because they are tired of the hours or the physical demands. Make certain that if a clinician is applying for the job of physician relations representative, it is for the right reasons. Make sure that he or she is committed to the needs of the position and not just the appeal of something different.

Anyone who is inexperienced in physician sales needs orientation and training. Clinicians must understand the organization's services from the perspective of the referring physician, and they will also need extensive sales training. Nonclinical staff need orientation to the clinical product lines and extensive exposure to the portals of access within healthcare. So the question of whether a clinical or nonclinical background is better is not answered by which is easiest. The best practices keep an open mind as they interview both types of candidates and then hire for fit.

## Special hospitals, special circumstances

When you are trying to forge relationships with specialists, a candidate with a clinical background is more compelling. His or her narrow focus, clinical depth, and understanding of the systems of access from within and outside the organization are an advantage. Someone with a clinical background is an asset at heart hospitals—where the representative is charged with working primarily with cardiologists, cardiothoracic surgeons, and vascular surgeons—and at some cancer centers.

Sometimes you can find good candidates within your facility, so it always makes sense to post the position internally and see whether there are individuals who indicate they are interested. Organizations are accustomed to posting positions on their Web sites and running ads in the local paper. Assuming you are doing the search yourself, ensure the ad clearly states the background you desire. Consider placing the ad under sales in addition to healthcare if your goal is to attract someone with strong sales skills.

If this kind of search works for you, that's great. However, many programs have recognized that the type of talent they are looking for may not be actively looking for a position. The best-practice organizations take a proactive approach, seeking good talent, sometimes at a national level, through word of mouth from market experts or at national meetings that physician relations representatives attend, such as those sponsored by the Forum for Healthcare Strategists, the American Association of Physician Liaisons, and the Society for Healthcare Strategy and Market Development. These organizations also have job postings on their Web sites. As with all proactive searches, word of mouth is a powerful tool, so use your network to learn who may be looking for a position.

## The interview and hiring process

The longer I was in a management role, the more humble I became about my ability to find the perfect candidate. The first several people that I hired were very good. As a result, I thought I was very good at finding the right talent. Then, I hired someone who became my not-so-subtle reminder that there is more to hiring sales talent than meets the eye. Experience and lots of work with some of the best in the business have given me insights into the hiring process and the tools the experts use to support the process.

**A Marketer's Guide to Physician Relations**

## Who should do interviews, and how should they be managed?

Like others within the facility, first-round interviews are managed by HR, through a paper screening for minimum qualifications. HR will generally do a follow-up phone interview and then ask the candidate to come to the facility for an on-site interview with the person who would be the candidate's immediate supervisor. All this is standard for most jobs within the organization.

If the hiring of sales talent is new to you, then be certain to take your time and do more interviews rather than fewer. Set up interviews with the chief medical officer or chief operating officer in your organization to assess how the candidate relates to those who spend the most time with physicians and clinical staff. When you schedule these interviews, provide the leader with a score sheet. On the sheet, list the desirable attributes and then ask the interviewer to score the candidate in each aspect on a scale of 1–5. It may also make sense to weight the attributes that you deem to be most important. Selling skills, for example, should rank higher than the ability to be a team player.

## Tools to support your hiring and implementation

There are several tools that can help you to hire the right person. Consider the following:

### Job descriptions

Good hiring always starts with concise obligations detailed in a job description. Although it's tempting to just throw something together, best-practice organizations take the time to really work through the job functions. Be specific, and make certain that the candidate knows exactly what will be expected of him or her. Spell out the percentage of time that will be spent on each function. This includes detailing how much time the candidate will spend in the field and on other activities. Most of the best-practice organizations recommend that the representative spend approximately 70%–75% of his or her time making face-to-face visits and creating field connections via physician-to-physician visits/educational events. The other 25%–30% is divided among other activities that may include setting appointments, planning sales calls, tracking and reporting, internal communications, and training. These elements are customized according to the environment, services, and program sophistication. Taking the time for all the little nuances and particulars ensures that the individual really understands what it takes to be effective in the role.

## Performance management tools

Organization leaders have long realized the significance of detailed expectations and measurable actions to assess performance. In the case of physician relations, at the time of hiring, the candidate should receive a list of performance expectations that specifies the baseline activities and results. Those individuals who come from a sales background—and especially those will receive an incentive compensation plan—will expect to see specific activity and outcome guidelines. HCA Continental Division's Riley incorporates an extensive description and review of the performance expectations during the interview process. "I go through the job descriptions and tell them their targets for the first quarter before I make the offer. I ask them: "Can you do this? Being straight right from the beginning is key."

At HCA Far West Division in Henderson, NV, Vicki Perfect, VP of HR, sets up a model that connects all the elements of the HR tool kit. Taking the time to create measures that are the right fit for the organization ensures consistency in HCA's model. Perfect and her team wanted to have specific operational actions that could be measured, including face-to-face appointments, meetings with the target physician and internal experts, connections with the target physicians via education events, and office staff relationship advancement. The management tool outlines the frequency of each activity. Depending on travel time and the number of individual physicians who are in the same practices, it is reasonable to suggest that the representative will complete 12–15 face-to-face appointments with a target physician each week. If there is strong opportunity to expand outreach activities within a new geographic region or there are several new physicians on staff, the organization will want to position frequent physician-to-physician meetings. As many as three per month is not uncommon in those scenarios.

Educational offerings are a wonderful way to connect physicians with your internal experts. Again, by detailing a specific number of events or activities, you provide the physician relations expert with a goal that seeks to advance the relationship and further the referral opportunities. This is the basic framework that is employed by many facilities that have strong physician management tools in place. Most organizations measure and report on their performance management on a quarterly basis along with a summary of their referral volume measurements. A report is produced to demonstrate the desired and actual activity and is tied to the results, measured in new referrals.

## Compensation

Best-practice organizations work hard to ensure that their compensation package is adequate to attract the right talent and achieve the growth goals of the program. This often starts with bringing representatives in at the right level and title, not because they will have a huge team reporting to them but because of the nature of the work and their contact with referring physicians. Money is never the only reason to take a job or the only reason to stay, but it does matter. The best people in the business are skilled because they have been nurtured and have grown within the organization. They have learned what makes it tick, and they have deep and strong relationships with the target physicians. The only way to retain this top-notch talent is to ensure that you reward them—and dollars are the most objective reward.

> *I think having a compensation program aligned with the results you are trying to get is key. At the end of the day, if you don't pay them to do what it is you're trying to get them to do, it's not going to work.*
>
> — Roger Smith, VP of HR, *HCA Continental Division*

Recent market surveys show the average starting salary for physician relations representatives to be $55,000 to $70,000. This is always a tough one because the dollar amount paid varies by market. Smaller rural communities or cities with a lower cost of living may be just below this average, while expensive communities will have a higher base. Representatives in some markets earn

**A Marketer's Guide to Physician Relations**

in the $40,000 range, and others earn more than $90,000. Remember that you get what you reward, and if you try to "hire cheap," you risk bringing in the wrong level of talent or you find yourself with a revolving door—training good staff only to see them move on for more dollars.

Although many healthcare facilities provide a base salary with merit pay and increases for inflation, recent interviews and studies show an increase in the number of organizations that have created a plan for performance-based compensation to reward those physician relations representatives who meet and exceed their activity and new-referral obligations. Many of the best-practice programs have worked closely with their HR leaders to provide support and create an approach that is consistent with their other incentive pay for executives and consistent with the culture of the organization. Although executive compensation often is measured annually, incentives for physician relations is more effective when done on a quarterly basis with their participation in the year-end bonus as a part of their fourth-quarter reward.

## Staff orientation

When a physician relations representative is hired for a new program, there is generally an all-out effort to get him or her out in the field talking with doctors. Organizations spend time working on logistics to support this effort. They provide laptops, car allowances, and target lists to the representatives. Orientations last from three weeks to three months.

For those who spend three weeks learning about their product, unless they have come from within the organization, there may be backlash because they do not understand the product as well as they should to sell it to physicians. Or, as they go into the field and begin to generate interest, the operations team tries to put on the brakes because they were prepared only for a little growth, and the new business pace is overwhelming.

In contrast, for those representatives who have a three-month in-house orientation, it can be a challenge to get them out and selling. They have settled into a routine; they enjoy the pace, the newfound learning, and the camaraderie of their new peer group. They sometimes struggle to really gear up for the field pace that is required.

If you have landed on either side of this, you can easily right the ship. It just takes awareness and getting back on track with a focused sales effort. There are all sorts of internal and external reasons why the orientation and initial field integration is created, so this is one of those times when you must get everyone on the same page, learn from it, don't expect perfection, and get on with implementing the program.

The bottom line is that a solid orientation for this role is essential. It is hard for the representative to stay focused if he or she does not understand what he or she is positioning. Equally important, you must make sure that there is a level of internal readiness to deliver. Those who keep their people field focused take the time to do so from the start. The individual who oversees sales must take the time to develop and oversee the orientation process. It should include internal meetings with key constituents to help the representatives learn clinical offerings, organizational culture, strategies for key service lines, operational and access processes, computer and database skills for reporting and tracking activities and outcomes and key message points that are consistent with overall marketing goals and objectives.

Unfortunately, it is not enough to schedule meetings for these dialogues. They have to be prepared in advance so that the internal team knows what you expect them to communicate with the new staff member. And the staff member should do some homework about each element of the orientation process prior to the meetings. He or she should come prepared with specific questions or scenarios to really learn what is needed before going into the field.

It's also important that the orientation includes sales training. Interviewing with some loyal physicians to gain perceptions during this orientation phase is another way to give the representative some field focus and hone his or her skills. Asking the new staff member to role-play discussions with referring physicians using the content they gathered during their orientation meetings also helps them to practice their sales skills while at the same time ensuring that they learned what they needed to learn before going into the field.

## Keeping staff on track

Everyone breathes a collective sigh of relief when the new representative is on board and ready to go into the field. And yet, managing even the best talent requires ongoing commitment and attention to the details of job performance.

Best-practice organizations maintain focus on the team's personal growth and skill development.

## *Involvement*

Although you should be careful not to waste the salesperson's talent on all the organization's issues, meetings, and processes, it is imperative to acculturate and actively involve him or her in the right way. It makes sense to have the salesperson feel like part of and understand the organization so that he or she can be passionate about it when going into the field. This can be done by carefully selecting which meetings representatives attend and when. Some organizations find that, rather than having them participate in a standing marketing meeting, it's more effective to ask the representative to attend a different medical staff meeting each month. Others will ask the representative to attend or present at a senior leadership meeting one or two times per year.

"Many staff that are in these roles are very interested in the greater good of the team; inclusiveness is important to them," says Terry Humphrey, an experienced marketer and physician sales expert who currently works for HCA Healthcare Corportation in Nashville. "What this means is that lack of inclusion in the team is a huge demotivator. Leaders need to find ways to have their physician relations staff involved internally within the realities of being in the field."

Involvement also means staying actively apprised of the changes in clinical services, technology, and quality outcomes. Develop a formal approach for the representative to spend one or two hours in service areas that have significant

**A Marketer's Guide to Physician Relations**

change, and always ask the representative to provide leadership with a brief that shares field intelligence and positioning strategies.

At Southeast Missouri Hospital in Cape Girardeau, Director of Business Development Don Fisher has a great system in place for doing this with his team. "We have directors or administrators come in and talk to us and bring us up to date as to what's happening," he explains. "Not only does it give my team more clinical depth, but it gives the service line directors more insight about what it is that we are doing. We have a two-way dialogue with my team asking good questions about the clinical piece as well as talking about what we need to do to for them. They know we have a genuine interest in seeing that service line succeed."

## *Participation*

There are two levels of participation. One is active participation with the program leader and other key leaders in the field efforts. The leader should go with the representative on field visits every two months. By spending a day with the representative, leaders can assess the representative's skills, increase their knowledge of key physician issues, and push the representative to reach a deeper understanding and to ask better questions. Those program managers who are intuitive will get a quick sense of the level of the relationships between the representative and physicians and also be able to assess whether the representative is able to push deeper or is stuck in a rut of more transactional, shallow sales efforts.

The other type of participation is when the representative arranges meetings between others from the organization and physicians and practices. This may include a member of the senior leadership, and often it can be another physician. When the top leader goes along, it is fair to ask whether there is a specific objective and expected outcome for the visit. Active participation in a site visit with a senior leader is the representative's chance to position his or her ability to advance the relationship. The leader has the right to expect more than just "howdy rounds." The leader should actively participate in the site visit and work with the representative to advance the relationship.

To create the right level and amount of participation, there needs to be active willingness and engagement by the leader in the discussion. The representative also needs to set the stage well for this type of visit. This kind of participation won't work if the visit is not adequately prepped or if it is conducted at the wrong stage in the relationship development process.

## Focus

We discussed focus at length in Chapter 1, but it bears repeating here that if the goal is to have someone in the field growing the referral base, then that's what that representative should do. Everyone at every level needs to resist the temptation to shift focus or use that representative for another role. The problems that referring physicians share with the representative have likely been around for a long time. The representative was not hired to create solutions or fix them but to work outside the facility to create relationships and earn opportunities for growth. The representative's obligation is to report

**A Marketer's Guide to Physician Relations**

what he or she learns, offer suggestions, create compelling reasons to consider the suggestions, and stay in the field doing the visits.

## *Personal growth*

Personal growth is important for most people. It's essential for someone in a relationship sales role. There is a constant desire to learn other/better/different ways to create an impact, to develop personal techniques, and to enhance background knowledge. The experts will tell you that to be effective in this role, salespeople must have three skills that are equally important: a deep knowledge of the product, an understanding of the internal process and packaging, and the ability to sell.

To be successful in the role, representatives must have a strong knowledge about the products they position. This doesn't mean they need all the answers, however. As a generalist, part of the key is to know what questions to ask and to identify who the right people are internally to get you the answers you need. Good product knowledge starts with a strong orientation, ongoing operational updates that are proactively initiated by the representative, and the ability to assimilate and learn what is most important and valued from the target referring physician.

In our work, the packaging is all about systems of access. Access breaks down to understanding the people who can get the information and get things done. Representatives need to know who the go-to people are when there is a problem or concern. They must be able to position how important a response is and communicate that to the right person internally. They also must understand the nuances of patient care. For example, they should know what tests are done prior to a certain procedure and what diagnosis is picked up at a primary care physician level and sent on to a specialist, versus the diagnosis that is uncovered and totally managed by a specialist. Understanding the package positions the representative as a valuable resource.

Understanding how to implement service-based sales with key stakeholders is the type of skill set that ensures that the representative gets appointments with the target physician and creates a strong dialogue that allows him or her to understand the physician's need and how the organization's products and services can meet that need. He or she understands how to close the meeting and advance the relationship toward closure. Good selling skills are a combination of the right mind-set and personality and a willingness to develop these aptitudes continually.

When I train physician relations representatives in a group, it's obvious that this comes more easily for some than for others. Some individuals are instinctual salespeople. For them, good training provides names for the different processes and helps them understand why there is a breakdown when one occurs. When I first began physician relations sales, one of the eye-opening experiences for me after participating in sales training was that by learning the process, I had an enhanced ability to self-assess and to understand what I needed to change or manage to enhance my relationships and earn the referral. There will be better results from the field staff if the training process is done by someone who understands service-based (versus product-based) sales, physician practice dynamics and how physicians make decisions.

**A Marketer's Guide to Physician Relations**

Good sales training is not a onetime deal; it should build on each subsequent session, getting more advanced and more in-depth with more product-specific scripting and interactive work. Ongoing learning is a good thing for all of us. But physician relations professionals seem to need it more than others. The desire to learn something new is part of what makes them tick. Those around them must prime the pump with new ideas to keep the energy alive.

## Sales management

The management of physician relations programs varies greatly by organization. And as the programs evolve, as the role and the staffs expand, there is an increase in the number of leaders who are accountable exclusively for this effort. When the sole focus is on physician relations (sometimes combined with other sales-oriented functions within the organization), there's more of a chance to be hands-on with the team. This supervisory role can challenge even those with the best skills, especially if the supervisor's management background has not included any sales oversight.

In working with new programs, I have found that these types of people generally do not totally fit in with the rest of the in-house team. The exact behaviors that we value when they are pushing along a referring physician or office manager can be seen as noncompliant when displayed within the organization. Leaders who have several other areas of responsibility in addition to physician sales should step back and create a plan and approach for reaching the program's goals, managing the representative, and keeping a happy middle ground of communication with internal stakeholders.

At HCA Continental Division, Riley's approach is to provide physician relations representatives with facts and data so they know what is expected and the tools they need to do their job. "It's tough enough without having resources to make their life easier," Riley says. "For example, remote access is key. I don't care if they sit at Starbucks and document what they have done or get the information they need. I make sure they have the technology to do their job. And then I honor their professionalism, give them goals, and touch base with them on a regular basis. I acknowledge that what they do is not easy, that it's really important and making a huge difference, and then I support them."

### *Reporting structure*

Physician relations programs are often organized under the business development or marketing function within healthcare organizations. Early on, if there is only one representative, he or she may report directly to the VP of business development. As the program grows, the organization might create a director or VP-level position that has oversight for all the field efforts, the tracking and targeting, and the internal integration. Having said that, however, there are many nuances to consider when evaluating the right reporting structure within your organization:

- **Leaders must have a good position of power.** This is more than just the right reporting level, although that is some of it. The program leadership must have the ear of senior leadership (assuming, of course, that they know how to use it), get attention when needed, and be able to manage things at their level when that is the appropriate option. At the onset

 **A Marketer's Guide to Physician Relations**

of a program, there is often a great deal of jockeying for control of the new position. That's good news because it shows that these departments feel they have a stake in the relationship with the physician. The key is to position this so that there can be the right attention and the right attributes to grow a focused program in the direction you desire.

- **Leaders must have a view of the top.** Back in the 1980s, when hospitals first hired liaisons to call on doctors (when the model and motivation were different than the current model), program leaders had little influence in the hierarchy. The reporting structure led to the demise of some programs. If the physician is important enough to have a full-time representative dedicated to him or her, then make certain that the representative has a very short conduit from the physician relations program to the top echelon of leadership.

Connection at the top helps with internal clout, too. When there is a VP in charge of physician relations, he or she generally reports directly to the CEO. Director-level staff also have a dotted line to the CEO for outward appearances and to make certain that others within the organization understand the importance of the physician relationship.

Every organization has some politics, and healthcare facilities are no exception. It is important to have enough internal impact to get the attention of other managers within the organization. This is about chain of command and having the power or clout you need when you need it.

## Reporting structures to avoid

There are some reporting structures that don't work as well as others. One of them is having the head of the physician relations program report to the VP of medical affairs or the chief medical officer. Although there are some outstanding and visionary chief medical officers, they are better suited to oversight of retention programs. Their focus is often on enhancing the internal environment for the physicians and for the patient-care experience. They are intent on fixing problems but not focused on the strategy side of growth.

Another structure to avoid is having physician relations report to the director of the hospital-owned practice network. Sometimes this can work if there is division between the clinic management and support team and the representatives, with a different manager and different staff to track and support the day-to-day operations. There should also be a distinction between each role. When it does not work as well is if the practice believes that the representative is also the one to complain to about the clinical operations or paychecks. When the representative takes on the troubleshooting and communication on a daily basis, it is hard to change hats and earn new referrals. This structure generally does not allow for a differentiation in the positioning approach.

In summary, the reporting structure generally falls under business development and/or marketing. But each organization must make the decision based on the people within its facility.

## Capable managers

Just as best-practice organizations need capable staff, so, too, do they need

     **A Marketer's Guide to Physician Relations**

capable management. Sales managers have a really hard time getting anyone within the organization to assess their job performance. With this checklist, at least they can do a self-check. As the number of physician relations programs grows, there is a tremendous opportunity for those who want to rise to the level of management. (Although I will refer to them as managers for the purposes of this section, "manager" is used simply to describe any person who has direct oversight for the field-based function.) Regardless of the program's maturity, effective leaders continue to balance their ability to look at the whole ladder, while never losing site of the individual rungs.

The manager's day comprises many parts that hopefully form a satisfactory work experience for the manager and for the team. The best managers have a range of abilities that form the right skill set for the role:

- They help staff establish the right habits and stick with them. Good work habits are the underpinning for any position, yet it is much different when you can actively monitor work performance in an office or a unit than out in the wild blue yonder. The best managers find creative methods and design systematic tools to keep apprised of their team's level of effectiveness in the field. They use tools such as performance management systems, weekly reports, ride-alongs, and field assessments to create a strong work environment. They trust their instincts in this area. If a representative is slacking off on appointments, they are comfortable confronting him or her even when lacking hard evidence. The approach and finesse that is required in this instance makes a real difference among strong physician relations leaders.

- They reward the positive. In a job that has a fair amount of rejection, the best managers find positives and recognize them. The world of working with gatekeepers, sitting in a practice for an hour only to have the doctor get called to deliver a baby or stepping out of the car in August heat and humidity is not glamorous. In addition, those who are good at their jobs add a full dose of pressure on themselves to keep up the pace.

- They recognize the positive attributes of their staff, and they do so in front of others. They put team members' names in their reports and call out members when members have a good idea or create inroads when others were unable to do so. Personal recognition goes a long ways on a day full of rejection in the field.

- They let people whine just a bit but continue to be proactive, as if to say, "Let's move on with what we can control—forward focus is the way to go."

- They keep the internal team on task and accountable to its obligations. The pace and the list of tasks on everyone's plate—including the operations staff—is significant. Even when there are great systems in place, there are times when the changes asked for by the physician relations team may get pushed to the back burner. With capable management, there are regular and systematic reminders, and there are documented expectations based on the internal communication plan. This is a tremendous motivator for physician relations staff, not because the staff

**A Marketer's Guide to Physician Relations**

expects that problems will always be fixed immediately but because the staff knows that there is someone who will bird-dog the issue and always go to bat for the staff's needs. The manager's accountability process naturally goes further than just making a call. Innate to the manager's ability to get things done is the ability to formalize and implement processes, which we'll talk more about in Chapter 6, and to track and report. The creation of systems is all about holding everyone accountable to do his or her part. And when others don't really understand the role of physician relations, then accountability needs to be even more objective.

- There are innovators who push themselves and the team further. What an awesome attribute for a physician relations leader to have. It is that blend of intuition and spark that lends itself to saying, "Let's try to position the orthopedic service with Dr. Smith this way and see if we can have an impact." It is the willingness to try a new approach to tracking or another way of looking at the integration plan with operations. It is not as though every idea is a magical success, but it does create wonderful synergy within the team. It creates market opportunity, even if only one out of every four ideas is a keeper. In the clutter of the market, that one idea may differentiate your services and cement a referral relationship. The part of innovation that separates great managers from the "all ideas, no substance" type is that the great manager has learned to share the idea, test it, gather feedback, and realize that beyond the idea there is a process for implementation that must be fine-tuned. The great manager also weighs cost versus benefit, so innovations are considered for their cost in terms of dollars and people and the benefits for the masses. In essence, we are talking about a strategic innovator.

- They create tools that demonstrate value. This is the attribute that is often the most obvious to people outside the department. Because the internal departments all have grids, outcomes, trended data, etc., they are interested in seeing if a "relationship program" can do the same. The best program leaders carefully think about the tools they need to be effective in creating the role, evaluating the role, reporting on barriers to success, and advancing the position. Some of today's tools are created to assess what is working internally, while others are designed to show the program impact. Most of the best program leaders with whom I have worked will quickly create preplanning, outcome, and issue reports. They balance measurement of activity in the field with the outcome and return on investment for the organization. With the ability to replicate the findings and report them out on a monthly basis, the best leaders use the database and other tools to more specifically home in on trends or market opportunities. Some do a wonderful job of showing the impact with graphs and charts in addition to using stories to show the personal side of the role.

- They make work fun. Of course, when you have oversight for a group of people who are gregarious, there is an almost mandatory obligation to lighten things up every now and again. Most field representatives are pushing hard to meet their weekly demands. The boss who can remind

**A Marketer's Guide to Physician Relations**

them they are valued, do something spontaneous, or make everyone laugh is a welcome addition to any management rank.

- They are straight shooters. Every bit as important as a little fun in the workday is the ability to know that if things are not going well with performance or with the ability to fulfill obligations, the leader must work to educate, demonstrate expectations, and critique behavior that is below the norm. The team appreciates that the leader requires adherence to baseline expectations not only for the field role but also for interactions and behaviors that are in keeping with the team's reputation.

- They have the right skills. First, let's address the way it is for many organizations that have physician relations reporting to marketing or business development: Many healthcare leaders have no sales experience. Rather, they tend to come up through operations. They will need to assimilate into a middle ground—between the comfort of how things are done within the facility and the external reality of what it will take to grow the referral base. Step one is awareness of this, step two is to really think about what that looks like and what tactical attributes help make it happen, and step three is having the desire to make that work. The other option is that we hire the right leaders by bringing in those candidates with a strong sales management background, which ensures that they have the sales capabilities. The essential skill is the ability to balance people issues and organizational needs. There regularly will be compelling needs that are gathered in the field, as well as from department leaders begging the relationship leaders to "go tell them about our new service." On both sides there needs to be careful management, the ability to ask good questions, to decide what fits with the strategic goals and what would be nice versus what is essential to address to earn more referrals. Both tactics have challenges. The expectation is that, regardless of the starting frame of reference, the right leader has the skills to create the right climate for success by working with both internal and external customer groups.

- They are willing to be held accountable. There are many positions within healthcare where it's assumed you are doing your part if people generally like you and you manage your budget. The leader who takes on the physician relations function needs to be comfortable with realizing that the program's success is measured by new growth. The leader is heavily judged on his or her ability to facilitate and manage this between internal constituents and the external team.

Certainly, many of these attributes are consistent with those you desire in every leader. Again, the difference here is that the physician relations role is relatively new to the healthcare environment, so there is a lot of internal misunderstanding about what is expected and how valued it is. The manager is the "face of the program" internally, so program positioning within the organization depends on how the manager carries the role.

© 2007 HCPro, Inc.   **A Marketer's Guide to Physician Relations**

# Leading effective team meetings

Most leaders are accustomed to leading meetings with their team. Although some of the preparation is consistent with the management of any other function, because the staff is only on-site for short bursts, it's important that the leader takes the time to prepare an agenda and maximize the limited time that the team is together. Most leaders have learned to prepare an agenda. There should be distinct areas of content, and it is the leader's obligation to manage the time allotted for each topic. If not, the meeting tends to get overrun with discussion about issues or problems.

A typical agenda for a for a physician relations team meeting might include:

- Information and updates
- Concerns and a status report on top referrers
- Product updates
- Skill development session
- Fieldwork and processes
- Shared discussion about trends

Every meeting needs to include something new and interesting, whether it's new ideas for messages, complete with a script and role-playing, information on technology, or a chance to have one of the team members lead a discussion on one of the selling skills. A change of pace keeps the staff engaged and interested.

Communication is a significant obligation for the program manager, in terms of both time and the number of groups and individuals with whom he or she needs to connect. Because of the nature of the physician's grapevine, the manager who spends more time working inside the organization than does the staff must discern what is new and what may have an impact on field communication. For physician relations representatives, there is frequently a "rub" because they feel like they are not in the loop regarding physician issues at the leadership level. It is the job of the leader to consistently remind the staff that it is rarely an issue of intentional omission when they are not provided with information and end up learning it in the field. Because this can be a never-ending battle, the obligation of the program leader is to encourage everyone to be proactive. In turn, he or she should work hard to create consistent methods of communicating new information to the field staff.

## Taking the team to new heights

The leader needs to both own the vision of the physician relations program's potential and be able to paint a clear path for ongoing development. With a strong visionary leader, the team can gain credibility within the organization, among the ranks of senior leadership, and—most important—in the eyes of the physicians served. The best leaders seek ways recognize and reward the efforts of those who are great in the field and mentor and support those who want to progress to the level of greatness.

**A Marketer's Guide to Physician Relations**

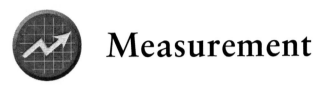

# Measurement

## The ROI of physician relations

Costs are up, reimbursements are down—even the public is taking notice
of the rising cost of healthcare. There are many reasons for the current cost
dilemma, but it's having an impact on the nation's hospitals in the same
way: They are under tremendous pressure to continue to grow in the most
cost-effective manner. Healthcare leaders are cautious about investing money
in programs and new employees to staff them. They want assurance that
the investment will increase usage and revenue. That's especially true with
programs such as physician relations that are outside the patient-care arena.
In that case, the organization's leaders want to make sure that the program's
benefits will substantially outweigh the program's cost.

Physician relations programs are growing in number and intensity in the market because they have the ability to meet leaders' expectations for a positive
return on investment (ROI). Hospitals have discovered that investing in these

programs and people can have a significant impact on referral growth in key areas. By carefully developing a measurement model, best-practice organizations clearly show how the representatives' interactions with physicians result in increased referrals and provide evidence of solid referral growth. It is clear method of demonstrating that this program was essential to making it happen.

Beyond doing what's right, those organizations that are willing to demonstrate their contribution to the bottom line are able to create good momentum for the physician relations program. (That's another best practice that we'll talk about later in the book.) This allows the organization to grow new business and add new physicians and gives these best-practice organizations new insight into how best to deliver care and be more competitive.

Measurement models also allow organizations to collect and analyze data and, based on the information, make adjustments and refinements to the program. There is nothing easy about setting up systems of measurement for physician relations programs. Best-practice organizations are usually blessed with one or more of the following attributes:

- They have access to good state data

- They're nimble enough to be able to create ways to extract the right data

- They're driven to measure data by the pressures related to the program

- They're experienced enough to have set up solid systems and tools that allow extraction of the right information to make the case

## Measuring for retention or growth

What we are able to measure depends on who we are targeting. Organizations that have found the loyalty and contentment waning among their most active medical staff members focus first and foremost on retaining existing business. Physician relations representatives create good customer service strategies and work to understand the doctors' concerns, to gain their involvement, and ultimately to enhance their satisfaction. If you are working with physicians who give you all the referrals they can, for example, your goal is to increase satisfaction, get them more involved, and stabilize or slightly increase their referral volumes as their business grows. It is a very important group, but since they are already giving you the bulk of their business, there's simply not much more to grow. Organizations with a retention strategy measure two main objectives:

- Physician satisfaction, including the number of issues or problems raised by the group of loyal referrers

- Volume of business, to ensure that there is no erosion and, if possible, some small amount of growth

Although many of the techniques in this book are helpful for organizations pursuing a retention strategy, our main focus is on those organizations that are engaged in physician relations as a growth strategy. For these organizations, the measure of success is new business in the door.

Best-practice organizations are intentional about using physician relations to earn new referrals. They target physicians who split their referrals between their facility and the competitor or those who do not currently send referrals their way but could. The goal is to use education and connections to encourage physicians to send patients to the facility.

To accomplish those goals successfully, best-practice organizations take the following actions:

- They determine to which competing organizations the target physician is sending patients

- They identify ways to differentiate their facility to earn these referrals

- They have the ability to track and measure whether the physician's referral volume has changed

- They make certain that they are working to grow the right kind of referrals

- They establish conservative metrics that all internal stakeholders agree show the program's contributions

 **A Marketer's Guide to Physician Relations**

Organizations with new physician relations programs generally rely on metrics or mathematical formulas to determine ROI. But best-practice organizations take the time to really understand the process for their facility. They glean market intelligence from the field and combine it with internal data and trends to get an accurate, detailed picture of the referral milieu. This process takes time and persistence to accomplish.

"The reality is that there needs to be a little leap of faith as organizations move forward with their sales measurements. The essential piece is to make sure that the organization is directionally correct and make sure not to let *perfect* get in the way of *good*," says Terry Humphrey, an experienced sales leader who now works for HCA Healthcare in Nashville.

## Using data to gauge results

To understand best-practice organizations' approach to measurement, it is valuable to understand their philosophy and technique for getting to the numbers. In Chapter 1, we discussed the need to grow the right business and to use data sources to understand the potential for growth clearly. From the measurement perspective, it's important to examine baseline contributions—to look at the before-and-after pictures, if you will. As you cull through the data, identify physicians to target for growth by starting with the strategic areas in which you have a strong potential to grow business and where you are certain you have specialists who are similarly motivated.

Once you have developed a target list, dissect each physician's individual referral contributions over the past three years to evaluate his or her personal growth trend. Some organizations like to count referrals only, generally recognized as inpatient encounters. Others look at revenue and volume for their inpatient encounters. Some measure inpatient and outpatient data, focusing the sales effort on a select group of diagnostic/testing procedures when there is a mixed portfolio. Each facility must decide for itself exactly what data it will measure. One caveat: Don't measure on revenue alone. The payer system within healthcare is extremely complex, and the physician relations representative has no control over reimbursement rates. The role of the representative is to encourage the physician to send patients—generally within a certain diagnostic category for starters and then across the continuum—to your facility. If that is your goal, that's what you should measure.

Once you decide what to measure, step back and dig into some of the data that will frame your measurement profile. The process is tedious but essential if you are going to establish clear targets and strong forecasts. The data includes the following:

- **Payer mix.** First, look at the current payer profile. Does the physician you are considering have the right mix to enhance your organization's profitability? Of course, I'm not saying you should turn patients away or refuse referrals because of poor payer mix. But if you are going to proactively encourage new business, you must evaluate this. Second, evaluate whether more business to your facility is feasible given the payer complement within the practice. If Dr. Smith is referring all of his

**A Marketer's Guide to Physician Relations**

patients to your hospital except for those covered by an insurance plan that you do not accept, there's probably not much room for growth from him.

- **Individual referral trends.** Although many facilities like to categorize physicians according to their practice group, it is important to evaluate the referral trends at the individual physician level. It's not safe to assume that they all follow one routine—even though the senior partner may sometimes tell you that they do! You should also determine whether there are splits within the individual physician's referral routines. If Dr. Smith, a family practice physician, sends a large number of patients to one hospital for cardiac care but only a handful of orthopedic cases, there's probably room for growth from this physician.

- **Physician demographics.** Evaluate demographics at the physician level. If Dr. Smith's patients all come from a geographic area that is closer to a competing facility, there may be room for some growth from the physician with the right approach from the physician relations representative. The forecast for this physician should be conservative.

Try to work with three years of trended data—or as close to three years as you can get. More data means a clearer picture of referral routines. This level of data scrubbing and analysis will give you the clearest sense of the ideal target and what type of referrals he or she may send your way.

Sue Pietrafeso, director of outreach programs at Sunrise Health Systems in Las Vegas, describes how her organization developed a measurement system. "When we initially started the program, our efforts to identify our target goals for sales were quite simple—it was all about market share. We didn't have a lot of depth of understanding at the time about the complexity of really understanding how to move the referral business until we got into it," she says. "So, for example, we would look at the trends for each of 25 cardiovascular surgeons in town and develop a projection around how much cardiovascular surgery business we could move based on that limited review. As we got more sophisticated, we started to recognize that we had to also look at the whole group and the dynamics those aspects would have and the accompanying strategies that would be needed to influence that level. What came to us after a few quarters was that sales efforts had to start further back in the referral chain than that—with the cardiologists, and even before that with internal medicine. All that has to be teased out as best as you can depending upon the data you have access to and really understanding where to gain influence and traction in redirecting existing referral patterns."

## Tracking primary care referrals

Collecting data about primary care physicians (PCP) is a significant challenge for many organizations because many do not adequately document their referrals to the specialists. They know the name of the cardiologist who referred the patient and the name of the hospitalist who admitted the patient but often fail to capture the name of the doctor whom the patient sees

 **A Marketer's Guide to Physician Relations**

regularly. It's likely the physician relations representative has spent years convincing this physician to refer patients to the cardiologist on your staff.

When organizations dig into this, they are amazed to see that their biggest referring physician is "none." This struggle has been further compounded by the rise in popularity of hospitalists. Best-practice organizations that employ hospitalists track, measure, and monitor the input of PCP information to their records.

Many organizations are staffed by private-practice hospitalist groups. In this case, such a mandate is a bit trickier to accomplish, and it falls back to admissions to gather information about the referring physician.

You can make a dramatic and immediate difference in your program if admissions consistently asks for and reports on the patient's PCP. From the standpoint of the physician relations representative, it is certainly much easier for the representative to visit a doctor when he or she can first evaluate a record of the type and number of patients he refers to your specialists for hospitalizations.

Those organizations that have a multilevel strategy spend time with the PCPs and "pull" the referrals through the specialists who use their facility. It is hard to create the pull if you are uncertain of the track record or the impact. Referral data not only benefits the physician relations program but also improves the quality of patient care. When patients return to their PCP, sending the physician a note indicating what occurred and the ongoing treatment needs not only improves physician satisfaction but also ensures the continuum of care.

"What the whole process of understanding the referral chain has done is changed the kind of dialogue my sales staff has with primary care physicians," Pietrafeso says. "Instead of going down the path of asking 'How does my hospital work for you?' we focus on 'Who do you refer to, how does it work, and why does that work for you?' We now more clearly understand it isn't just one piece but the entire referral spectrum that must be influenced to see change. And the team now has physician relationship diversity so they can fully appreciate the needs and sensitivities of all of the participants in the referral process."

## Gather market insights from the field

Data is one way to evaluate the best targets and to create accurate forecasts. The other vital component is the market insights gleaned from field intelligence. Once the field representatives have created a list of potential targets, best-practice organizations use anecdotal information from the field to cull it.

For example, an organization might remove a target from the list because he or she has a close relationship with someone on the board of a competing hospital or there is a quality or safety concern. They might decide to tread carefully with a target because of political concerns or because the physician has had a poor experience with your facility in the past or might cause friction with one of your other physicians. They might put a question mark next to a

 **A Marketer's Guide to Physician Relations**

physician about whom little is known. And, finally, they would of course go forward with those physicians who are desirable to the organization.

So who makes these assessments and on what grounds? Some of the very best lists are the result of a one-hour meeting with the top few members of the leadership team. If the leaders have been in the community for a long time and are willing to look over the list, this is a great approach for streamlining. For some facilities, members of the C-suite are the best resource for this task.

Although it's difficult to get them all in the same room at one time, most will be willing to peruse a list and offer insight if they know the physicians. The chief medical officer or vice president (VP) of medical affairs is another good resource. Those who have come up through the ranks and have long-standing relationships through the entire medical community are invaluable in steering the physician relations representative in the right direction. It's most important to tap these sources for the physicians who are not practicing at your facility, since it's not likely you have a lot of intelligence on them. Obviously, it is easier when they are splitting business because you have quality indicators and peer review to support the opinion of those who give input.

Long term, the most effective approach for gathering information is to glean the details from the physician relations record once regular visits have begun and the physician is in the database. The representative will know how quickly the physician tends to make changes, what the physician's current referral patterns are, and the physician's conditions for making a transition. Regardless of the source, layering the solid trended data with the intuitive market intelligence makes for a more fully developed target list and the opportunity for better forecasting of results.

## Strategy for forecasting

Best-practice organizations work hard to create accurate forecasts for estimating volume potential as a result of the physician relations program. They understand that although it is not an exact science, the methodical planning and predictive process can make a real difference. Forecasting offers the following benefits:

- **It forces preplanning.** The process of creating a forecast allows the internal team to evaluate past market trends, detail expected changes, and predict the future.

- **It sets realistic expectations for the team and for leaders.** Physician relations representatives perform better when they are accountable for specific results. Reality is a very healthy manager. Likewise, leaders benefit from seeing up front what they can expect to garner as a result of the physician relations effort.

- **It stimulates internal communications.** The forecast allows those services that are targeted for growth to step back and evaluate the capacity and their ability to manage the impact of growth. They are also given fair warning that they will need to provide the tools that will help the representatives build relationships with the referring physicians, such as clinical outcomes data and time for physicians and leaders to go

**A Marketer's Guide to Physician Relations**

with the representative and share details about the service. The forecast defines the agenda and spells out how much growth is anticipated. It is also a good reminder that there must be focused effort on this service and the field function for that to happen. It is a delicate reminder of the intent for the relationship strategy.

- **It gives leaders validation for their support of the effort.** The forecast reminds leaders that there is real dollar value in the program and that the program leaders are willing to commit proactively to an outcome. In an environment where dollars are tight and outcomes often imprecise, there is great value in the ability to predict and to meet those predictions.

Forecasts should be done yearly, when the business plan and targets are updated. On a quarterly basis for the first year or two, the representative and his or her leader may wish to tweak it. I am a strong proponent of not allowing too much overhaul—tweak is the operative word here—unless there are major, unanticipated market changes. There are two reasons for this. First, it is possible to overplan, which robs the representative of time in the field. Second, some sly physician relations representatives will never leave it alone and keep trying to "play" the forecast purely for purposes of their incentive-compensation advantage.

## *Forecasting techniques*

There are several different approaches and methods for forecasting. Again, the exact formula isn't the most important thing—rather it is about finding a sound method that will work for your organization.

Forecasting is a mathematical model that relies on historical data and those variables (e.g., referral patterns) that you believe you can change. The forecast should be driven by trended data at the physician level. The market variable is intelligence based on past visits from the representative. (If the forecast is for a brand-new program, there will be no strong field intelligence and, thus, is little more than just a good guess. That doesn't mean you can't or shouldn't go through the process, however.)

It's a good idea to walk through the forecasting process in great detail. That way, when you go to do the actual measurement, the formulas are in place, and it becomes a straightforward mathematical computation.

Here's the suggested model for when you have solid admitting data at the individual physician level:

1. Start with your target list of physicians and your desired areas for growth.

2. Look at revenue and volume numbers for the last three years for each individual physician level. Predict what his or her overall revenue and volume would be with no change.

3. Document any market changes that are likely to occur and predict, based on the methodology of the CFO, the impact.

4. Use that information to determine the baseline number of expected growth for each physician without sales.

5. Hone in on revenue and volume numbers in the strategic areas you are targeting. Check to see if they are in keeping with the physician's overall trend. Make adjustments if needed.

6. Based on the annual percentage of assumed growth and the variables (items 3–5), estimate the percentage of growth potential. List it both as a percent and as an actual number of referrals.

One caveat: If you are unable to track PCP referrals accurately but you are aware that you will be using visits with the PCPs to increase their awareness and ultimately referrals into a specific physician group/service line, this can be accounted for in the forecast. If you are a small facility with only one or two specialists, it works to just increase their referrals by a larger percentage to note your impact on the overall referral market. If you are a large hospital/academic medical center and assume that there will be many specialists in the department or section who benefit from the physician relations program, look at an overall section total that is larger than the individual forecast numbers add up to be. This might sound tedious, but if each representative is focused on a group of 250 or so physicians and this is an annual exercise, perhaps that puts it in perspective. It is much easier to stay focused on advancing the relationship when you know exactly how much of an impact you are projected to have on the referral numbers.

Ed Dougherty, the VP of physician network development at Lehigh Valley Hospital in Bethlehem, PA, worked with Program Director Nancy Heacock to demonstrate the ROI for their physician sales effort. They have refined the data of measure each year, but they started with gaps in the primary care data. After full analysis, Dougherty determined that it was "comparably muddy data." But it was a starting point, and a forecast in the early stages, for most healthcare facilities, is a tool to focus the effort and estimate the potential. Take Dougherty's advice, and be careful of "analysis paralysis" when it comes to forecasting.

## Activity measures

Most facilities measure activity in addition to results. Many weight each one so that 60%–70% of the performance management tool weighs results with the remainder giving credit for the ability to meet or exceed the activity measures. The weight for the results needs to be proportionate to the confidence in the data to measure it. And many start with a much higher activity weight because they can measure it and because it encourages consistent field activity, which, after all, drives results.

Nonsales healthcare experts sometimes debate the validity of rewarding a physician relations representative for activity—in other words, as they see it, for "just doing their job." They argue that every job includes tasks that

**A Marketer's Guide to Physician Relations**

are necessary to accomplish the main goals of the job and that setting up a meeting is not worthy of rewards for excellent performance or for incentive compensation. But today's representatives face significant challenges when attempting to get face-to-face visits with physicians in their offices. Some offices ban representatives altogether.

Pharmaceutical companies hire the best and the brightest salespeople to enhance communication and make connections with physicians. As healthcare facilities follow suit and flood the practices with more and more represent-atives, it's only going to get more difficult to schedule a meeting and have quality time with a physician. As competition for face time increases, a few things will happen:

- Those who do not bring value to the physician and his or her staff will not be invited back

- Those who say they are there to learn about the physician's needs but who simply tell and sell will be first to lose their slots

- Programs will need to make certain they consolidate their impact on practices, so those facilities that have a large number of service-specific representatives calling on the same physician will need to rethink their tactics

- Some will say, "We tried a physician relations program, and it did not work"

With so much market turbulence, those representatives who have stayed focused on solid messages, a strong work ethic, good techniques, bringing value, and staying consistent will be rewarded with the opportunity to make an adequate number of appointments per week. And those who are actively involved in supporting their efforts believe strongly that the activity should be measured.

So how do you measure it? Best-practice organizations have worked hard to make the model, method, and measures very clear and easy to understand. "At the end of the week or the end of the month, people are going to look at the combination of how many practices did we touch as an initial barometer and in how many practices did we do something that could impact positive change in our direction," Dougherty says. "From my experience in sales, I know there is a correlation between the amount of activity and revenue. Activity leads to results. It would have been unnatural to attempt to have a program without some metrics, so we decided to measure both activity and revenue to start, and although we started with heavier emphasis on the activity side, we now weight 65%–75% of what we accomplish on the actual outcomes. And our outcomes targets will change depending upon the hospital and the market area and medical staff associated with each."

The measurement of activity relies heavily on careful assessment of the types of activities that are known to grow the referral base and the careful definition of those actions. The most common activity measure is the number of face-to-face appointments with targeted physicians per week. Nationally, the average for this is about 12–15 visits per week.

**A Marketer's Guide to Physician Relations**

When counting the number of appointments, pay careful attention to the criteria of an appointment. Remember, these appointments are not easy to get, and salespeople do see the world from their own angle, so make certain that you clarify what an appointment is and what it is not. For example:

- It is not an appointment with the physician if you see only the office staff

- It is an appointment if you come with a plan for your time together, which includes actions and expectations for the meeting and closure to a next step

- It is not an appointment if you catch Dr. Smith in the parking garage and ask how things are going

- It is an appointment if you arrange for Dr. Smith to meet with the cancer center director about advancing their referrals to this service area

Beyond the number of face-to-face visits, other common measures include physician-to-physician meetings, meetings with office staff, physician attendance at a suggested continuing medical education (CME) or other education event, and physician participation in a medical staff event/special meeting. The trick here is to find things that are known to encourage the target physician to learn more or relate more to your organization and the physicians who practice there.

For the majority of your activities, select categories that can be sustained for a minimum of a year. The next step, again, is to again clarify what counts in each of the categories. Define the criteria as tightly as you can. Then, assign a suggested frequency to the activity. You can determine how many times per month or per quarter you expect the activity to occur. For the representative, this detail creates the road map of activity that needs to be integrated into their sales plan—the tactical action plan for their target physicians.

With this level of detail, a good representative should be able to map out his or her daily and weekly tasks, to accomplish the desired activity. If they are accomplishing all these activities, if they are the right people for the role, and if they have been given products and services that are right for the market, then their only obligation for ensuring results is a solid plan for advancing the relationships through messages and differentiation. (We'll talk about that more in the chapter on differentiation.)

## Tracking activity and results

The tracking of activity and the integration of results continue to be areas of interest for many programs—old and new alike. They are all seeking the best, most efficient way to track results and to have the kind of reports that demonstrate the impact for senior leadership.

Best-practice organizations have a system to track their activity and results. Some organizations build them internally, while others purchase and customize contact management systems. As the interest in physician relations grows,

**A Marketer's Guide to Physician Relations**

database companies are introducing more and better products. Developing a tracking system is not just about acquiring the right software, notes Allison McCarthy, principal of Barlow/McCarthy in West Dennis, MA. The software is a tool and not a magic bullet. The actual performance success of any tool depends on how its functionality and customization effectively document the relationship process and outcomes.

Physician relations professionals all too often select software without thinking about their overall process. In the end, they're dissatisfied because the system or tool doesn't flow naturally into their day-to-day functions or achieve their desired objectives. To avoid this problem, ask the following questions in the early stages of development:

- What information must be captured?

- What other system has this information (e.g., credentialing, recruitment, finance, etc.) that we could integrate into the tracking system?

- What information do we need to collect from the field?

- What does the system need to do (e.g., maintain calendars or integrate with existing calendar functions, integrate with organizational e-mail systems, document physician meeting discussions, assign next steps, track sales plans and implementation progress, trend physician responses to survey questions, capture and trend issue resolution)?

- How will staff access the system (e.g., through laptops or PDAs, via the Internet or remote server access)?

In addition, consider the types of lists and reports that should be routinely generated:

- Targets by specialty, credentialed versus noncredentialed, ZIP code, competing hospital status, etc.

- Qualitative feedback on important trends or issues, such as results from one-on-one discussions with a target physician group about the reasons for its steep decline in referral volume

- Sales staff performance reports, including number and type of visits conducted, CME sessions arranged, and hospital orientations provided, measured against performance expectations

- Activity reports that demonstrate the sales efforts made on a target group of physicians so that a side-by-side assessment with referral volume, revenue, and contribution margin trends can be made to determine the cause-and-effect relationship of the effort

An organization that has multiple marketing or promotional tactics working in tandem creates the most powerful marketing message. In these advanced programs, other functions also may be integrated with the tracking system. Examples include:

**A Marketer's Guide to Physician Relations**

- Documentation of marketing communication efforts that show which physicians received a direct mail piece, for example, so that representatives can reinforce the message in their face-to-face meetings

- Interface with other areas of the physician strategy, such as physician recruitment, so that the physician relations team can use information on a physician candidate to build and implement their retention strategy with that physician

- Integration with the call center so that representatives can use the information captured by your physician-to-physician line to assess the effectiveness of the referral made as well as encourage additional referrals to that service

Beyond these factors, other aspects must be considered, including the size of the physician relations program, its budget, the computer literacy of the staff, and the organization's security concerns.

With all that preparation in place, the organization is now well positioned to select a software tool to meet its needs. Through this preliminary planning work, the hospital, health system, or clinic can identify the software program that will be the best fit, versus having the tool drive what information is collected and reported. Although many organizations choose vendor-hosted tracking software or systems, there are still many that develop homegrown systems to track their physician relations initiatives.

OhioHealth, a multihospital organization in Columbus, OH, developed a unique contact management system three years ago that meets the needs of its sophisticated physician relations department. Kurt Stull, director of physician relations, and Troy Miller, manager of strategic planning at OhioHealth, built the system based on specific requests from stakeholders. "We wanted to combine a physician database with an off-the-shelf contact management system and an issue-resolution system. No such software or technology with those parameters existed," says Stull.

Previously, OhioHealth had an access-based contact management system and had built issue resolution functionality through the hospital's Lotus Notes system. However, those functionalities did not interface and were ineffective.

"Through our homegrown system, we have these various pots of information that can now 'talk' to each other," says Stull. "We have the ability to collect physician profiles and, at the same time, record physician visits and issue-resolution information."

Stull says the advantages of developing a homegrown system include flexibility, full customization, and a central repository for information that can be accessed by anyone with a username and password for the system. In the case of OhioHealth, Stull says they have encountered no disadvantages during their experience. "However, organizations have to commit to making this successful, to respond when needed, [and to] provide the manpower and budget commitment that's necessary in maintaining the system," he says.

**A Marketer's Guide to Physician Relations**

Regardless of your organization's size and physician relations goals, tracking capabilities are essential in demonstrating the value of those efforts to that entity. The organization can then make informed decisions about how this tactical approach fits into the broader mix of hospital-physician strategies and which efforts are yielding the best results.

# ROI, measurement models, and methods

Measuring the impact of a physician relations effort is the result of many parts of the infrastructure coming together. Assuming you are confident that the physician relations team is at or above its activity targets, this should translate into measurable new referrals—that's the goal, right? The consistent theme among all the best practices is that they measure impact. All have a method of providing quantitative outcomes, and they monitor change. They collect the field intelligence and study success in the form of growth or flat and declining volumes, as an indication of the need for a change of course. Having said that, the outcomes measures that are currently employed by best-practice organizations are as innovative as their leaders. In the simplest terms, the measurement models today are broken into two different types—physician-specific and service-line.

## *Physician-specific impact*

A physician-specific measurement model is certainly the most logical, the easiest to justify, and the most straightforward. It is the way to go, as long as your organization does a good job of capturing the name of the primary and referring physicians.

At the beginning of the year, the organization analyzes data and develops the forecasts. The growth forecast, including the rationale behind it, is shared with key members of the leadership team—most notably the CFO. The internal stakeholders agree which physicians to target and how much "credit" the physician relations team will get for results. It is crucial to determine this last point up-front. Negotiating for it after the fact is always disheartening if you have a financial leader who is skeptical of the impact of your program. He or she will make all sorts of excuses and give all kinds of reasons for the increase that have nothing to do with the program.

The moral of the story is that you must preplan. Put a stake in the ground about what you will produce and how you will demonstrate results. The next step is to work with the IT team to create a special quarterly report that shows revenue and volume changes for the target group. As part of this report, it is also good to look at overall trends in the strategic service areas. The physician relations team may need to adapt the plan to make sure that the organization is getting the right growth in the right direction overall—it's all part of being a team player and being proactive.

Finally, evaluate the actual quarterly data against trended numbers and the forecasts. Report this information to leadership alongside the activity report. Include information about any new physicians you have added, along with data about their referrals.

At the end of this process, you'll want to determine whether you need to adapt the field efforts for the next quarter. Some programs look at the data

**A Marketer's Guide to Physician Relations**

monthly, which is great if you can get it and use it. The cautionary note, of course, is that splitter growth can have some immediate results, but the work that is done with new business rarely shows results so quickly. Concentrate on the overall trend rather than feeling high or low every time the program experiences a little blip.

Michael Thomas, VP of strategic planning and marketing at East Texas (Tyler) Medical Center Regional Healthcare System, prefers monthly updates. "We review every referral by every doctor in our employed groups," he says. "We know which doctor sent what business to each specific destination. But beyond this analysis, an important difference is that we also look at referral patterns by physician. It's about working to understand through the data where you have a chance to change a referral."

## Service-line trends

For many organizations, the breakdown in this method occurs because they have their representative focused heavily on the primary care community and they cannot effectively track their admissions. Organizations that have three to four strong service lines that they are promoting might just measure those specialists. The built-in assumption is that the representative pulls the referral from the PCP through the specialist to the facility.

Others do some forecasting and evaluation at the physician-specific level, especially to help motivate and coach the physician relations representatives to meet their growth obligations, but rather than use the physician-specific data as the ultimate measure, they opt for a service-specific model. When programs are in the start-up phase or when they are internally at odds about whether to trust the data, the next best option is to focus on growth in the target service lines. The way this works is that new business is measured in the top three to five service lines that the physician relations team has been asked to focus on for growth.

As you get further out from measuring the actual interaction, there are a few more challenges. The first is trying to figure out what growth within the service line should be attributed to this effort. This is a concern of other organization members that the physician relations program will get more credit than it deserves. Some are conflicted about the fact that a generalist physician relations representative will have an impact on many other services because of the relationship and consistent presence in the office, so the program does not get all the credit it should.

Responding to those who question whether the physician relations program is responsible for growth: There is never a perfect answer for the source of every single referral. In fact, changes may be the result of several different events or messages that resonate together. But, in the case of this effort, we also know that many of those other messages and events were in place long before the sales effort, so their contributions should already be a part of the mix.

Again, the method for creating program measures is to look at past patterns and then to compare and give credit. It must be negotiated on the front end. If there are other new and different happenings that contribute, negotiate that also. For example, the cardiac service line has been growing by 25 cases each

**A Marketer's Guide to Physician Relations**

year for the last three years. We assume that with the addition of our new EP physician, we will double that volume even with nothing being done.

With this discussion and the projection, then the physician relations program will measure and take credit for growth this year that is more than 50 new cases. It becomes clear that for some organizations, there needs to be a great deal of negotiation. Taking a conservative approach and clearly defining the contributors on the front end can go a long way in saving you from the measurement blues on the back end.

So, how do we reply to the representative who says, "If we only measure these three to four service lines, all the good work we are doing to be responsive to the needs of the practice outside the scope of these areas goes unnoticed, or at least isn't credited to us."

To overcome this challenge, some have opted to add some anecdotal commentary to their reports, calling out the areas where the representatives have been focused, telling stories, or documenting specific physician changes. Others will look at the service lines but also take partial credit for overall growth—much harder to negotiate with some CFOs—and still others will assume that if they are growing cardiac, they are also going to see increases in pulmonary and rehab programs. In this case, they just state assumed overflow credit without putting an actual number to it.

The challenge of exactness and allocating credit in measurement is twofold. There is getting credit for the program, which we have discussed. But the bigger challenge occurs when incentive compensation for the representative is reliant on these measures. Assuming that you have come to terms with all of the naysayers, here's how to set up this approach:

1. Look at the trended data in the top three or four strategic service areas that you have targeted for growth. As part of your data analysis, evaluate the specialists who are contributing and at what level, explore which ZIP codes the business comes from, and determine any "external factors" that may influence the service growth over the next year. This might include additions or retirement of a specialist, changes in managed care, the competitor campus across the street, etc.

2. Determine how much growth is expected based on past trends. Consider any variables that will affect this growth, and present a projected growth number for the service.

3. The measurement process is similar to the physician-specific model in that, on a quarterly basis, you will ask for a service-line report that shows new referrals.

4. If you have added new physicians to the service as a result of the physician relations effort, it is also appropriate to track and measure the new physicians on board.

5. Although the measurement report is on total service lines, the program leadership needs to dissect the data at the physician level to understand how the growth occurred and to adapt as needed.

    **A Marketer's Guide to Physician Relations**

The easiest part of the measurement is the analysis. The challenges seem to come with getting the rules set up internally, ensuring that the right data is reported in a timely manner, and managing the physician relations representatives who have a tremendous desire to make certain they get credit for everything they feel they deserve.

At the end of the day, none of the models are perfect. Joe Paine, the CEO of CHRISTUS Schumpert in Shreveport, LA, has a refreshing slant on this issue: If there is growth occurring, he says, the last thing we should do is to fight with each other over who should get credit for it. Rather, focus on the real opportunity, which lies in replicating the success and working to grow even more.

## A measurement snake pit to avoid

Sometimes service-line leaders will step forward with their budgets and ask the physician sales representative to project the line's growth potential as a part of budgeted dollars. Base your projections on data trends, market variables, and field intelligence. Don't fall into the trap set by their saying they are budgeted to grow 10% and they need you to contribute 5% of that. (Physician relations' 5% will of course be the *second* half of the 10% growth projected, so the internal team will get the credit if there is 5% growth only.)

Proceed with eyes wide open, and clearly understand and question, if necessary, the factors they considered in their growth projections. Often the 10% is based on how much the organization needs to spend rather than on tangible actions. It seems like the smartest approach to look at the actual numbers and then work to negotiate how much of the service-line's budgeted numbers the program can contribute, as well as how there will be tracking and results reporting for them.

## How do you share the results, and how often?

Good reports are of no value if they are not understood or not shared with the right stakeholders in the right context. Best-practice organizations understand the value of a quality report, and they find ways to showcase their program and the impact that physician relations has within their organization.

### *Departmental activity reports*
The program should look at activity reports on a weekly basis. If a representative falls behind in the desired number of visits, then an additional previsit planning report is in order. Obviously, there is a need to assess whether the issue is time management, inability to get the appointments, too few targets, or a lack of understanding about how many calls it takes to get more than the baseline number of appointments. With a previsit worksheet, the leader can work with the representative to make certain that they are able to get all their calls scheduled. The weekly activity summary does not have to be formal. The leader just needs to see whether calls are being made, to whom, and with what objective. And if a tracking system is in place, these summaries can be generated easily.

**A Marketer's Guide to Physician Relations**

## Monthly and quarterly summary reports

Program leaders generally provide the senior leadership with an end-of-the-month summary. The most effective format I found is a one-page summary that includes a quarterly summary of new referrals or of revenue and volume, generally demonstrated in year-over-year comparisons. The rest of the report is the same monthly and quarterly activity, including the total number of field visits, the percent of visits to each targeted physician type, and key topics for strategic messages to each. Include market intelligence from the field and a summary of the top complaints that the representatives hear from their target physicians. Some also create a line graph to track and trend the top issues.

Finally, include strategic services/key messages or targets planned for the following month. Including next actions will, from time to time, trigger a leader to share additional information on the topic with the representative if the leader knows the rep plans to have it as a central message point. The report is short and easy to understand. Leaders can read it quickly and feel in touch. And it allows an opportunity for senior leadership team members to ask questions and delve deeper.

Reporting the quantitative results is best done with a breakdown of key categories and a roundup of totals. Charts and graphs that visually detail forecasts versus actual results or trends and impact are always informative. Those who are the best at measurement are often the most focused on generating awesome results. It's your opportunity to put the physician relations team in a position to prove its success.

# Pushing the envelope

As programs mature in their ability to measure those things important to assessing sales impact, they will begin to search out more advanced tracking and monitoring methods. To enhance activity reporting, many programs begin to break out sales activity by service line. This permits one to assess whether sales resources are being appropriately allocated based on the organization's strategic goals and objectives. Not all service lines are created equal, and therefore it is important to assess periodically whether sales is supporting those areas deemed to offer the greatest growth potential. If the organization's strategic plan calls out cardiovascular and oncology as key growth areas for the year, then sales should focus more effort and resources in these areas. Breaking out sales activity by service line provides a quick check that resources are being directed into the appropriate areas and in the right amount.

Another common sales activity breakout is retention versus growth. For those programs that have both target groups, breaking out sales activity into these categories provides another quick check on whether the program is slipping back into heavy retention instead of focusing resources on growth opportunities. Both of these activity breakouts can be monitored on a monthly basis along with overall sales activity, but at the very least they should be evaluated quarterly so that midterm adjustments can be made if necessary to keep the program on track and aligned with the organizational goals for the year. As discussed previously, making or exceeding forecasts is the true measure of program success.

**A Marketer's Guide to Physician Relations**

Some sales programs take an extra step to show their impact on growth by comparing volume among their targeted physicians to a comparable group of non-targeted physicians. In statistical lingo, this is similar to setting up a control group or, in the case of drug testing, a placebo group. In this case, sales resources are directed toward the targeted group of physicians, and no resources are directed to the non-targeted group.

For this comparison to be meaningful, it should be done by service line or physician specialty. Here's how it works: Let's say that the organization identifies cardiology as a strategic service line for the coming year. As a result, sales targets cardiologists believed to offer the greatest growth potential and directs resources and field visits toward this group. When it comes time to measure results, volume growth of the targeted group is compared with all other cardiologists who were not targeted by sales. If the growth on a percentage basis of your targeted group is greater than your nontargeted group, then that's a good indication that sales had a positive impact.

Of course, as with any approach, there are limitations. Your nontargeted group consists primarily of physicians with low growth potential by design; however, one can argue that at least some of the above-average growth is the result of sales and would not have occurred without the effort. Finally, some programs are actively engaged in measuring the holy grail of marketing and sales—namely, a measure of the financial ROI. Most industries, including healthcare, have struggled with this issue from the beginning of time. The basic problem is that it is extremely difficult to identify cause and effect when it comes to sales and marketing. Did the patient come to your facility because he or she saw your TV advertisement, or because a neighbor highly recommended you?

The inability to determine cause and effect is one of the reasons why direct marketing and sales campaigns have become so popular in recent years. When someone responds to a direct marketing campaign, you know that the interest was sparked by the campaign, so most CFOs have no problem attributing any dollars associated with that customer to your marketing effort. You also generally know what it cost to execute the campaign, so you have what you need to measure ROI (gain/cost).

I know we all wish measurement was that easy with physician relations. It's not, but there are still some ways to do it. Regardless of the methodology employed, the most important step is reaching some type of agreement with the CFO prior to determining what portion of growth will be attributed or credited to sales. This will always be a negotiation process based on assumptions that are agreeable to all the parties involved. Some have elected to compare volume growth in your targeted physician group to a group of nontargeted physicians in the same specialty.

As we discussed earlier, the nontargeted group serves as a control group. If cardiology volume increased 10% among your targeted physicians and only 5% among nontargeted cardiologists, then sales should be credited with some portion of the growth.

This is where your agreement with the CFO comes into play. If the CFO has agreed to credit sales with half the incremental growth, then some type of average contribution margin for cardiology cases is applied to this volume, and you suddenly have the gain attributed to sales.

While many hospitals still struggle with accurate cost accounting, at the very least your annual budget identifies direct costs of the sales programs, and most organizations have some method of allocating indirect costs to departments. Now you have the cost component, and ROI simply becomes the financial gain achieved against the cost to achieve this gain. Although not a perfect solution, many other industries don't get much closer to a true measure of ROI than this.

And, of course, we have the whole question of how to account for growth in outpatient services and its contribution to sales ROI. Few programs to date have fully incorporated the outpatient component, although those attempting to do so are using the same principles described above for the inpatient setting.

## Using measurement to enhance the program

The organizations that continue to push forward and look for more, better, and different ways to grow their programs and enhance their own growth are those that dissect their measures and constantly look for better ways to use the data and better ways to do the job.

Like them, you can look through the different reports and ask yourself some of these tough questions to determine whether there is more that can be done to enhance the physician relations effort. Ask the following questions:

- Are representatives getting in the door and having good dialogue with physicians but not getting new business?

- Do the same issues stay on the report month after month?

- Are the representatives learning field intelligence that we can better harness to position our competitive advantage?

- Have we hit a plateau with our growth trends?

**A Marketer's Guide to Physician Relations**

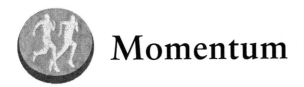

# Momentum

## Capturing the elusive essence of momentum

The barriers to starting a physician relations program are low. And most organizations with new programs quickly pick the low-hanging fruit. Best-practice organizations make the physician relations or sales effort an integral part of their strategy to expand the breadth and depth of services. They use the program to shore up market changes, to prepare markets when there will be new facilities, or to keep the dialogue going when hospital-physician relations turn rocky.

Up until this point in the book, the best-practice attributes have all been quite tangible and very businesslike, but momentum is a little harder to get your arms around. Does momentum come after you hire a certain number of new physician relations representatives? Is it built on a 15% increase in revenue and volume for your oncology program in the third quarter?

Momentum might be sparked by actions and successes, but there is more to it than that. It is also about having a team that is energized and passionate, that spreads its enthusiasm when working with the practices.

Momentum is that capacity for progressive development and the power to increase or develop at an ever-growing pace. It is forward movement, in both a physical and the psychological sense. When an outsider looks at physician relations programs with strong momentum, there is an instinctual and very focused way that they operate.

It is possible to replicate many of the process elements and emotional charges that lead to results for these best-practice organizations. It starts with evaluating the attributes and understanding the mechanics of creating momentum for your program. Best-practice organizations that have really captured the momentum know it is made up of concrete action and that energetic feeling. You see it in their approach—even in how they cheerfully respond to an age-old complaint from a grumpy physician. You see it in how leaders work to find options and alternatives when a service is at capacity so that they don't have to turn patients away.

Part of the essence of momentum is a can-do attitude. But momentum is not just high emotion or people doing the right thing (although all of that is good and contributes). There are tangible physical signs of momentum.

Best-practice organizations that have momentum on their side share some common characteristics. For starters, they demonstrate an environment that recognizes change. Program momentum is often accompanied by three hospitalwide attributes as well.

### Strong desire to measure results

East Texas Medical Center (ETMC) is one of two regional referral centers in Tyler, TX. The community is served by three independent cardiology groups, and both tertiary facilities are interested in having as many cardiology patients admitted to their facility as possible. The sense was that ETMC was not getting the quantity of cardiac referrals that was proportionate to their primary care base. So, as is appropriate when faced with a change in momentum, Vice President (VP) of Strategic Planning and Marketing Michael Thomas started with the data.

Early last year, he dug deep into the referral patterns for each physician at an individual level, working to determine the nuances, including referrals, their origins, the payer mix, and the overall numbers. He extracted some troubling findings about the status of the organization's cardiac referrals into the cardiac group. Many originated from ETMC–owned practices, yet the patients were admitted to the competing facility.

The leadership team set about addressing the issue; the senior leaders initiated talks with the whole group and individual members. The group was resistant. Although the data got some traction for the hospital, real change occurred as a result of proactive communication from the group's referring physician base. Physicians in ETMC's medical staff office wrote letters to the cardiac group sharing their preference for hospitalization of patients whom they were referring to the group. The letters indicated that if the cardiac group didn't change its referral pattern, the physicians would start sending their patients elsewhere. Indeed, volumes fell for the group until they made a change. Admitting volumes are now up 30%—a significant increase. It was gutsy, had a powerful impact, and successfully shifted momentum. Thomas started with data and ended with data. There was a strong desire to shift the results and clear evidence that it happened.

### Strong marketing messages for physicians

> "The business is changing and is so fluid that there is always something new and different that we are trying to sell and to get excited about."
>
> — David Flicek, senior VP of clinic operations, *Avera McKennan Hospital & University Health Center, Sioux Falls, SD*

Program momentum is aided by the ability to state clearly what is a fact and to be honest and forthright. Program momentum comes about because everyone knows where they stand. The approach and method of accomplishing this is certainly customized to the style and approach of leadership.

Generally, while we're focused on momentum of the program, we realize that there is evidence of strong management with a commitment to pushing the program further. At the program level, there are specific markers that indicate a program is pushing forward and looking for better and more innovative ways to grow the referral base.

**A Marketer's Guide to Physician Relations**

Susan Milford, vice president, strategic marketing and planning at Centegra
Health System in Crystal Lake, IL, started her physician relations effort within
the cancer service line. "The accredited cancer center gave us the opportunity
to develop a new approach to marketing within the organization," she says.
"The marketing initiative for that area gave us the opportunity to stretch the
organization a bit into physician relations. It took a fairly short time of having
a physician salesperson for us to show some results."

## The ability to grow new business

The number-one sign that there is strong momentum is sales success. This is
first and foremost measured in the ability to forecast new referrals and then
to meet or exceed those expectations. Taking this a step beyond, we see a
growth that is steady and consistent and, long after the low-hanging fruit is
plucked, the programs continue to add to their relationships and gain new
referrals. Milford puts it best: "The single most important driver of momentum
is results," she says. Sales success also takes the form of increased market
presence in a geographic area. Those programs that harness momentum then
see market share shifting in pockets. Part of this may be coming from some
solid branding by the organization. This feeds through the practice as patient's
step forward asking about a specific facility. Couple this with a physician
relations representative focused on imparting the details, and the referral
process is complete.

Physicians, like consumers, want to be "part of the group." If everyone knows
that Ace Hospital is the "best" for cancer care, it is then momentum that gives

the organization the chance to leverage that market presence for additional growth. Momentum facilitates new growth even with the physician as we observe one office staff member tell another about a positive referral experience with an organization. The same does occur (although not as often as we would like) with one physician in a group telling another one about a positive experience. Unfortunately, any negative experience is shared even more readily, with a negative impact on momentum.

James Wente, president and CEO at Southeast Missouri Medical Center in Cape Girardeau, MO, saw this firsthand in an organization that is big, unique, and diverse. "Obviously, in an organization with our size (2,000 employees), we can't expect everyone to know each other, including the medical staff," he says. "But we have hired many new specialists, and this has given us the opportunity to rethink how we introduce those new physicians with those who are already a part of the organization. By doing these introductions, it gave the medical staff the opportunity to interact with each other more than they normally would . . . it got them talking. And what it demonstrated to us is that we don't make this happen behind a desk but out there in the community."

If you currently are enjoying program momentum, consider ways to sustain and build on it. Communication is certainly a foundational part of this. Milford agrees that the first measure of momentum is business growth. For her, gaining momentum is intentional, with solid planning and good internal communication. Talking to her about her future plans, and about the tools and techniques she uses to gain internal buy-in, and listening to her innovative ideas, one can tell that the pace and energy will continue. It is her purposeful communication with the physician relations and marketing teams, with senior leadership, and with the operations teams that creates the right level of buy-in to grow referral relations to the next level.

## *Program development and growth*

Another outward sign of good momentum is the growth that occurs within a program. This can take the form of physical growth, such as increasing numbers of representatives, additional geographic range, services that are part of the physician relations team's accountability, or growth in internal visibility and credibility.

Most programs start with a minimum number of representatives. Everyone is reluctant to add full-time staff until they know how the program will work. With one or two representatives, decisions are made to either limit the number of physicians in the target pool and know that some will just not get visits (preferred) or give the representative all 500-plus doctors that the representative will be able to visit once a year (a strategy that can be maintained, but that's not so good for growth).

The next logical step is to look at the impact and the reach and to consider additional representatives. This assumes that there are enough physicians who could be targeted to justify additional staff and that the internal capabilities are up to the task of caring for more referrals if they are generated. It also assumes that the first representative has proven his or her value and demonstrated the return on investment.

Leaders will need to assess the timing of this and the cost versus the benefit. There is no perfect time to add members to the team, but often it occurs when there is a good, strong uptick in referral volumes. Innately, the message then becomes, "If one can get us all of this, just imagine the impact if we were to have two representatives." Use the internal momentum, demonstrate the impact with numbers, and move for expansion as soon as the time is right.

## Geographic expansion

For some organizations, momentum takes the form of geographic expansion. Assuming that there are adequate specialist/faculty relationships, the desire is to expand the geographic reach. Of course, this often requires more staff and always demands better systems of access, but regionalization of the program and the enthusiasm surrounding the new market opportunity is a definite momentum builder, so momentum feeds more of the same.

At CHRISTUS Schumpert Health System in Shreveport, LA, the outreach effort expanded from a 50-mile radius to a 150- to 200-mile radius. "We did that through educational opportunities, introducing ourselves to administrators, case managers, and emergency crews, so it's not just physician relations activities," says Lori Marshall, regional director of physician development and sales. "It's really about helping with issues in the community."

## Service augmentation

For some programs, the momentum is visible when the representatives are asked to represent more and varied service capabilities. This is most evident

**A Marketer's Guide to Physician Relations**

when special programs that are originally kept outside the purview of the relationship team get included.

### *Increased internal credibility*

It is very exciting and a sure sign of momentum when there is more active involvement of the representatives at a strategic level within the organization. This takes the form of:

- Leadership seeking out the feedback or input from the representative

- Responsiveness or inquiries in regard to reports generated by the team

- Requests for presentations or input from the representatives

- Interest and willing support from department leaders

- More talk about physician growth topics

Program credibility must be earned and happens slowly. It is important not to confuse the initial intrigue and enthusiasm with credibility and long-term, sustainable momentum. The initial sizzle simply gives programs the opportunity to position the messages, reports, and tools that become the infrastructure for gaining the traction within the organization. With these programs, the position and momentum is important not for political clout and prestige but to ensure that there are solid mechanisms to support the relationship efforts internally, once they are created externally.

Within most facilities, there are one or two leaders on the team who are not certain that the program is all it's cracked up to be. They become believers when you can offer proof in the form of new referrals and when they see that physicians are using and appreciating the representative's connection. As they see the upside, they also relax in the knowledge that there is limited downside for them. Consider the chief medical officer who is concerned because he or she thinks physician relations should be part of his scope of responsibility. Once he or she is able to see that their relationships are actually enhanced and that he or she is getting better field intelligence, he or she often become a more active supporter. Good momentum develops when the internal team feels the program is credible, adds value, and gets the right results.

At Columbus (OH) Children's Hospital, VP of Market Development and Promotion Donna Teach attributes much of the organization's success to having the right internal champion. "No physician relations professional can implement any of this without a very strong, high-level physician champion, whether that's your medical director or chief medical officer," she says. "You cannot implement this without one person championing it, and that person has to be very high in the organization to be able to perform broad-scale change."

## Expert positioning

Momentum occurs in two different ways. Sometimes there are forces that give energy, lift, and excitement to something, which is often what I see with new program development. I call that the golden child era. The momentum just flows, and there is recognition for each referral victory. The buzz is alive. But we all know that no department, product, or person can be that golden

 **A Marketer's Guide to Physician Relations**

child forever. Enjoy the halo while it lasts, but create a plan for momentum moving forward. Foundational to making this happen is the program's expert positioning. Remember that TV ad tagline, "When E.F. Hutton talks, people listen"? That is the expert positioning for the program within the organization. So how do you get it? By offering objective, timely, and meaningful information that demonstrates that you are an expert. And, by the way, you lose the advantage in a heartbeat if you pretend to be an expert in something you are not. The key is to carve out the niche area of expertise and use the power and information very wisely.

> *Our physician relations effort demonstrated results with ample evidence that they had doubled the volume on our referrals. With that proof, there was no question that the team had the expertise to advise us on how to achieve more of that—in which service lines and in what specific markets.*
> — Joe Paine, CEO, *CHRISTUS Schumpert Health System*

# Momentum and the competitive personality

Many hospitals develop physician relations programs because their competitors are strong, determined, and agile. This contributes to more challenges in trying to grow the referral base. Some organizations approach the physician with an optimistic attitude. They encourage physicians to step forward—no request is bad, and they consider all ideas. The challenge of this approach, of course, is that many of the requests simply cannot be fulfilled. Yet the willingness to look into it, to explore and to share the rationale for a yes or a no answer, ensures goodwill in the marketplace. If enough desires are fulfilled, there is hope in every request.

For those who have significant competition, this is a huge momentum challenge. David Flicek, senior vice president of clinic operations at Avera McKennan Hospital and University Health Center in Sioux Falls, SD is advancing the organization's clinical offerings. "First, we started with liver transplantation, and [we] are now looking at bone marrow transplantation," he says. "Those types of services tap the resources of the whole campus. The whole campus has to step up to deliver those services effectively—pathology, nursing, infectious disease. These kinds of efforts raise the level of performance of the entire organization. From that perspective, it constantly pushes us to be cutting-edge."

Control of this level of momentum is obviously bigger than a physician relations program. So, within this setting, the underdog program role must be to facilitate messages both ways and to create opportunities for the facility to be seen as "can do." Getting to that level is a victory as it reduces the market position for competing facilities.

## Motivation comes from satisfaction

There is nothing better for momentum than having a truly satisfied customer—be that the internal leadership team, the referring physician, or your specialists and hospitalists. Best-practice organizations want to repeat their successes, so they learn as much about the needs of their customer and their product to find ways to really enhance the level of satisfaction. It's a powerful self-fulfilling approach that many of the best practices have harnessed for success.

Another aspect of satisfaction is the ability to keep good physician talent. If the job has the right rewards—and money is part but not all of it—then there is likelihood that you will see enhanced retention. Because when physicians are satisfied with the world experience and the culture, they create a good environment for themselves and for the others they work with.

All of us have heard the statistics about turnover in the work force and the numbers of unhappy workers. In my experience, this job would be dreadfully difficult if you did not feel a level of satisfaction and a role in the program's momentum moving forward.

Avera McKennan has an elaborate physician compensation system, customized to different physicians and different locations. You might think that this would create distress and dissention, but it has achieved the opposite. "We have less than a 2% turnover rate—we have very loyal physicians to the system. When I bring in a new specialist to the system, the physicians don't complain that they have to split the pie with someone else. They trust us and know we are going to do right by them. And having that buy-in as a baseline makes the business growth strategy so much easier to accomplish," says Flicek.

## Creativity and innovation

At best-practice programs, program interest and momentum is generated as a result of creativity—finding new, different, and innovative ways to enhance referral opportunities. This can include lots of little and not-so-little changes to the status quo. For example:

- Find new clinical data to showcase your efficiencies and outcomes in cardiology

- Use a long-standing social event as the platform for getting to know the new members of the medical community

- Create incentives for family practices to encourage those who use hospitalists to come to your campus

Creative ideas give you opportunities to connect. When these are dovetailed with a visit strategy, they create good synergy—both for the target physicians and for the organization. Beth Israel Deaconess Medical Center in Boston employs a tool kit with a variety of benefits that can be offered to referring

**A Marketer's Guide to Physician Relations**

physicians that helps tie their referrals to the organization and, more importantly, is offered to them based on what those referring physicians say they need. This tool kit includes a clinical information system that links the tertiary specialist, the community physician, and the patient in a three-way interface. It also includes a contracting vehicle that gives individual and small groups of community physicians the ability to join in and take advantage of managed care contracting size.

Beth Israel also provides more than 100 continuing medical education programs across eastern Massachusetts per year. Elaine Monico, director of network development at Beth Israel, says that her team is integrally involved in those efforts. "We open the door and are always scanning the market trying to locate attractive groups to talk to and present one or more of our offerings as a way to extend the hand of tertiary-community relationships," she says.

It goes without saying that using creativity is not a typical healthcare phenomenon. That means the stage must be set to communicate internally that there is a need for trial and error with ideas and suggestions. Those who do it well have created a method of communicating this internally and a culture of tolerance for new ideas.

The bigger venue of creativity is innovation—that ability to define and deliver on a process that takes your program to the next level. Oftentimes it falls to the leader, so he or she is able to keep the representatives in the field. Although creative ideas can generate short-lived momentum and interest, it is the innovation that creates a surge of momentum for the program.

As I look at it, innovation is the great idea surrounded by the right analysis, process, and planning to sustain change. The best-practice programs create innovative approaches to manage competitive threats, to position new and clearly differentiated services, and to augment methods of earning new referrals through the sharing of clinical outcomes.

The service recovery program at Columbus Children's Hospital is an example of an innovative program that creates momentum. "We actively communicated to practices that if you encounter a situation where you are experiencing long wait times, or triaging of your requests and you're ready to send the referral elsewhere, you should give me a phone call," says Teach.

"Give me a chance to make it right. Give me a chance to help you get what you need and to recover that referral. So basically before you pick up the phone and refer them somewhere else, please call me. Even if I can't do anything about it, I want to know about it. Usually it's a communication issue. So the liaisons can then follow up directly with the product line and see if there's something that can be done with the wait time," she says. "If they really feel like the wait time they have been given is not appropriate for the acuity of that referral, then it gives us an opportunity to make it right."

Is it really a good thing to tinker with what is already working? Obviously, we are working to create positive energy for the program. Creative and innovative change is the right thing to do when there is a window of opportunity. Equally important is to stay with the basics. Create a sound strategy, pay

**A Marketer's Guide to Physician Relations**

attention to all the basics, and put out the right effort for success. Then look for opportunities to augment and enhance what is working and keep all the parties interested by sharing what is new, interesting, and relevant for them.

## Can you be a best practice without momentum?

It is rare that facilities have every one of the best practices operating at peak performance. But you cannot be a best practice if you do not have the ability to self-assess and to create and sustain momentum for your program long term. So while it is difficult to evaluate momentum, if you even question whether you have it, then it may be time to go back to the strategy, look at the people and how communication is disseminated, and consider opportunities to innovate and enhance the relationship and the outcomes. If you have it, you probably know it.

When in doubt, ask yourself these questions, and you will know if it is time to get inspired and freshen up the approach.

1. Do the representatives seem to be "in a rut" with identical routines each week?

2. Have you tried new, different ways to share clinical outcomes in the last quarter?

3. How many times do the physicians call the representative to ask questions? (Calling to present a problem does not count.)

4. How many times in the past year have you created a new approach that required research, buy-in, and a process, and then implemented it with shared results? Although finding an innovative solution to a problem is great, don't count those solutions that were just to fix something broken in the market.

 **A Marketer's Guide to Physician Relations**

# Planned integration

## Picture of a collaborative organization

Physician relations is not an island unto itself. The best practices are aligned and integrated with other key service areas. They collaborate with planning, marketing, physician recruitment, and the medical staff office. This can take the form of a structural requirement or a communication strategy. Many organizations, as they shift to service lines for implementation, work to integrate the sales effort to ensure synergy and constancy of message.

Whenever I hear physician relations leaders say that they have perfect relationships with all other services, departments, and people, I think of Lake Wobegon, the fictitious boyhood home of public radio's Garrison Keillor, where "the women are strong, the men are good looking, and all the children are above average." Although many programs wish it were so, and some departments are solidly integrated with others, the ability to stay in sync with all the services on an ongoing basis is not easy to achieve. And it never happens without proactive effort.

Each of us likely has experienced strong collaborative relationships, both as a user of a product and as a provider. What a welcome experience when there is that synergy. Our ability to work better together internally creates a better outcome for the physicians—both those with whom we work and those we have targeted. At the most fundamental level, it shows itself in reliable messages, consistent implementation, enhanced intelligence, and better outcomes. It would be great to have every department and service integrated in their physician relationship approach, but it doesn't take total integration to make the cut as a best practice. Some areas make a difference, where there are rewards for the strides taken to develop collaborative tools, including data experts (planning or decision support), marking, and operations.

Clearly, integration with planning is internally driven, as it assists us in forming a strategic approach to the model and tells us the impact. Integration with marketing and communications and operations has an impact on the delivery of our messages and ultimately the delivery of patient care. It is essential that we provide consistent messages and ensure that our messages match what we provide. The operations part is a no-brainer; there must be the ability to deliver on the promise, and the promise must be at the right level to ensure consistent delivery.

**A Marketer's Guide to Physician Relations**

# Integration with data experts

The planning function takes different departmental forms depending on your organization. Whether this is your strategic marketing team, decision support, finance, or a planning and business development function, it's integration with the department that has accountability for strategic planning, defining target demographics, strategic services for growth, segmenting the market and creating the business plan. And more important, it's the group that has access to most of the data physician relations programs need to target their efforts, produce forecasts, and measure outcomes.

Programs that demonstrate consistent growth over time have a very intentional plan in place. They take a long look ahead and have a methodical style to gain the right kind of business from physicians with the best potential. Planners and decision support team members are recognized for their logic. It makes for good credibility with the others internally if it is the planning team that is front and center in detailing the market opportunity, analyzing market potential, and determining the key services to position. They are creating lists based on trends, not emotion. They are not choosing services based on market enthusiasm but rather on growth opportunity, reimbursement, and contribution margin.

Emotion comes as much from those who are not in the field as from those who are. Say the chief operating officer (COO) hears that there is discontent in the ranks of cardiology at a competing hospital. If there is no plan in place and no ability to extract the data and analyze the market potential, the impulse is to send the physician relations representative running to snatch all those cardiologists. In an environment without a plan, there is a great deal of chasing shiny things, but there's limited consistent working of prospective referral sources, and much of those who are chosen are there because of a hunch or because it feels good.

With a plan in place, there certainly will be the flexibility to "test" that group, but there will be strong, planned referral opportunities as well. The right mix is weighted toward planned sales efforts while also providing the ability to respond quickly to unforeseen opportunities as they arise. Along a similar vein, there is potential to slant the data or the focus within the program. Having a neutral and objective party to collaborate on the strategy, target services, and the demographic targets can go a long way toward making sure the program has sustainable goals.

Frankly, I have seen times when a pet project of an individual leader results in encouraging the internal team to grow something that, although nice, is not validated by the data. Although it may be an isolated instance, it is much less common when the decision support team is actively assisting with the plan. Recognizing that any direct sales effort, including physician relations, is a very expensive strategy, it makes sense to have a global evaluation by a credible source.

The only way to get these things is to have an ongoing relationship with a planner, and the planner rarely if ever approaches the physician relations team. This is about internal sales. The physician relations team serves itself well to

 **A Marketer's Guide to Physician Relations**

seek out the expertise of the planning team members and to find ways to make it easier for the planning team to help the physician relations team.

Working with data experts has the obvious advantages of data integrity, as discussed. There can be consistent processes, including timely updates and data evaluation and regular summary reports.

Working with the decision support team/planners, the leader of physician relations can do a yearly update of the business plan, which includes strategic growth areas and the physician targets. As programs evolve, there is an opportunity to synthesize the hospital data with the field intelligence to create a solid targeting approach. We've already established that perfect data is probably not a reality, but enhanced data to improve field success is absolutely a possibility with this relationship.

Whether the referral outcomes are tracked directly by the decision support staff or the finance areas, the planning team generally has access to it. For some best-practice environments that collaborate with these planners, they receive a quarterly referral update. In some states, if the data is available, they are also able to evaluate the competitive shifts. Florida is one such state where the type of state data, which is generally communicated by the planner, provides an excellent picture of the market changes.

Last but not least, in some markets, the decision support and planning experts are the most tuned in to legislative issues. For states with certificate of need or those fighting malpractice battles, there is great benefit from learning about political issues that will have an impact on the physician's everyday world.

Active business planning with the decision support experts, marketing, and physician relations—generally led by a vice president (VP) of business development—is a wonderful catalyst for innovation and also for practical discussion about relationship-building strategies and communication with physicians. When implemented, there is great opportunity for joint sharing of all the different views of the physician growth perspective.

At Centegra Health System, Susan Milford, vice president of strategic marketing and planning, regularly hosts retreats to motivate teams to work together. The retreat begins with the different groups sharing information and then moves into a planning phase, which allows for interaction. The model is to ask "what if" rather than to create a document that says how things are and how the group wants them to be. It's a great way to consider the possibilities.

In the same way, whether through a retreat, internal meetings, or regular written updates, both physician relations and marketing communication have an obligation to serve as the strategic data arm between the field representatives and planning, communicating feedback from the field representatives to planning. This may take the form of physician feedback about a product and service receptiveness and responsiveness. If there is an interest in more or different technology, new expertise, new delivery methods, or even new research options, this should be shared.

 **A Marketer's Guide to Physician Relations**

# Integration with marketing

Marketing is a word with multiple meanings. You hear people talk about "marketing their products" or "marketing their physicians," often via activities that seem to be sales or pseudo sales. To do it justice, we have to talk about how we are using the term marketing and how its integration occurs with physician relations.

"A healthcare organization has many publics that it must influence to accomplish the organization's mission," says Larry Margolis, president and chief marketing officer of Storandt Pann Margolis in LaGrange, IL. "Marketing is key to impacting the actions of any of those audiences, especially physicians, as hospitals are trying harder than ever to align with this group. Not unlike the clinical integration of medical care, the integration of marketing and the communications to all audiences is critical to achieving organizational objectives. Physician relations is simply a marketing function as we use a mix of tools from product design, communications, and distribution to affect buying behavior."

In healthcare organizations, the strategic level of marketing creates the path, defines the marketing strategy, creates the implementation plan, and serves as "communication central." In our view of the physician as our customer, marketing is the broader process, and physician relations becomes the "feet for marketing" in creating messages and identifying specific opportunities.

Some organizations have sales and marketing working in different departments from very different agendas. This occurs when marketing is focused almost exclusively on promotion and that promotion is geared toward the consumer. Equally as often, the physician relations program is set up as an insulated entity. There are many reasons for this, including turf wars, personality conflicts, competence issues, and workload distribution.

If this is your situation, evaluate the benefits of collaboration and then take the first step. In some organizations, marketing and physician relations must fight for the same share of the budget and recognition from leadership and other internal stakeholders. In others, there is simply no perceived need for the two groups to work together. Again, if the physician relations team can find synergies in messages, branding development, or the delivery of clinical capabilities, the team should step forward and begin building relationships.

There are many organizations where marketing and physician relations report to different people, but they still work together. When this is in place, there is generally a more advanced approach to physician marketing, often evidenced through shared Web strategies, a call center integrated with marketing, or some referral development calls to action that pull through practices.

Many best-practice programs have a shared reporting structure, with both physician relations and marketing reporting to the same VP. This structure obviously makes synergy easier because the people in both departments are around each other and because they often function off a shared plan. As a result, these programs have a consistent branding strategy for both consumers and physicians that is supported by consistent key messages and a similar look and feel in their marketing brochures, collateral materials, Web content, and other marketing tools.

This is the case at Centegra. "One of the key strategies when you're looking at marketing overall is sales," says Milford. "Knowing your customers and who's bringing you business is critical. I believe sales is the key strategy of the overall marketing plan. As such, we operate in teams in a matrix format. We have the overall marketing plan, and then we have priority service lines. So there is a team for cardiac, cancer, ortho, etc. Communication is vital, for it acts as a continuous way to reeducate the team about how the components all work together in tandem. When I first structured things in this way, in early 2000, maybe 25% of the programs were structured like this. Now the tide seems to be turning, and it probably is more like 60%–70% of the physician relations programs are integrated organizationally within marketing."

Integration really matters. Frankly, it requires a willingness to take the plunge and create the relationship if one does not already exist. In the early days of physician relations programs, there was a bit of a rub with many marketing departments. The early physician relations departments existed autonomously and often implemented marketing communication functions for physicians. This structure still works sometimes, but there are vulnerabilities, including mixed messages from different areas, planning that would replicate some areas of interest and leave out others, and financial economies of scale. Certainly those drawbacks are enough motivation to admit that working together has advantages—if not for the departments, then surely for the organization overall.

Integration is more important than ever. The marketplace for hearing and retaining messages is absolutely cluttered. So, the ability to identify needs and position benefits is complex and challenging.

Working with physicians, there is a very real obligation to create clear, distinct, and consistent messages. We are in a time when physicians have more and more choice and control. It all means we need to have a plan; we need to be consistent in how we live the brand, and we need to communicate our key messages over and over again. Best-practice organizations always start with the plan and their process of creating the right approach from the marketing tool kit—those elements that are part of the marketing mix.

## The marketing plan

For healthcare organizations, the physician is both someone we create marketing about and someone we market to. Marketing that features the expertise of an individual physician or a physician group and encourages patients to use the physician or physician group's services is an important consumer strategy. It also positions the organization as the provider of choice for the physician and the consumer.

The physician relations effort aligns more fully with those marketing efforts that seek to grow business from the physician. And as we work to earn referrals from physicians, there are many elements within the marketing mix that can support and advance the relationship. The starting point is always the marketing plan.

In Milford's model, the marketing manager is responsible for doing the analysis and writing the plan, including the sales component. Once that is developed, she brings the team together to review and further clarify the plan. When plans are developed, creating an inclusive process that allows the physician relations team the ability to plug in and share strategies is essential. If it is done in collaboration, there can be good attention to communication and involvement for all the physicians. Some will receive personal visits, others may receive direct mail updates; careful planning will ensure that the right tool is used to provide a message of interest to each segment of the physician community.

Just as there are several components of the marketing tool kit to consider as you establish your plan for physician growth, there are several methods that organizations employ in each of the following areas to enhance the physician relationship:

**Research.** Numbers sell in healthcare. As we work with physicians, the ability to use numbers to demonstrate the impact of our efforts is a powerful tool. Memorial Health University Medical Center, Inc., in Savannah, GA, has done quite a bit of analysis to help get the physicians on board.

For example, says Vice President of Regional Development and Sales Don E. Tomberlin Sr., Memorial created a correlation coefficient on physician-to-physician visits to demonstrate a positive return on investment (ROI) of the time specialists spent meeting with referral sources. "Physicians are scientists; they love data," Tomberlin says. "Eighty-five percent of their decisions are based on lab values, so we develop our own sort of lab values from this correlation coefficient that they really responded to." If you need to have physician support, there is value in taking the time to do the research and presenting it the way a researcher would.

**Web.** Many organizations have portals to communicate directly to the physician. As well, the Web has become a powerful tool for streamlining patient access, giving physicians the ability to track their patients via an electronic medical record from the comfort of their own offices. Talk about a marketing tool! Geisinger Health System in Danville, PA, had great results with this.

"It not only helped our referring physicians, but it was a tremendous benefit to our own physicians as way to send information back to the referring physician," says Kathy Dean, Geisinger's VP of marketing communications. "At the end of the night, the information automatically prints out in their offices—no more snail mail. And once we had a few of our physicians buy into the benefits of this program, they became our champions for selling it internally to the rest of the medical staff."

**Direct mail, fax, or in-house mailings.** There is a tremendous opportunity to connect with physicians on topics of interest, as long as it is relevant and to the point. Columbus (OH) Children's Hospital uses a physician update packet. VP of Market Development and Promotion Donna Teach says it was created out of necessity. With so many departments trying to send information to the physicians, there were mailings going out all the time. Marketing stepped forward and offered to create and manage the packets. Talk about a win-win.

 **A Marketer's Guide to Physician Relations**

It is more cost-effective, and because the practices now recognize that the packet is a valuable source of updates, the physicians are reading them.

Geisinger uses a similar tool called Fast Fact, which has become the company's staple for sending updates and timely information to physicians. This one-page sheet also has a companion note card that can be direct mailed to reinforce or to expand the reach when necessary. "We have it in both electronic and print format because different doctors want to access it in different ways," says Dean. For this best-practice organization, sending information in the format that each physician prefers is an important element in physician relations communications.

Another option is to enhance existing tools by personalizing them with the interests of the physicians in mind. Make a statement with those things that you need to make sure the physician sees. This may include an invitation to a CME event, advance notice of an upcoming consumer promotion, or a specialty-specific referral guide. Direct mail won't get attention simply because it arrives in the mail—it must be created in a purposeful manner. And don't send mailings so frequently that they'll end up being ignored.

The newsletter has long been a communication staple with the medical staff. Organizations have gone through ups and downs with it as they continue to fine-tune the tool to match the needs of today's environment. Best-practice organizations employ several options, such as a full newsletter that offers in-depth clinical updates from a medical writer, shorter news briefs, or a combination of both. What works best in your market really depends on the preferences of your medical community—ask them and they will tell you what they want.

**Marketing communication tools.** The physician relations team often needs to help traditional healthcare marketers as they determine the right marketing communication pieces. The pace of a practice does not allow time for the physician to sit and read brochures after the representative leaves. This is especially true if the piece speaks to multiple audiences (e.g., patients, families, consumers, and the physician). If the team is looking for a "sell sheet" or a leave-behind that has impact, provide relevant up-to-date clinical outcomes and easy access, even if internal physicians and specialists think you should be sending out slick "chest pounders." Some physicians, will be annoyed if you waste money on slick communications. They'd rather you spend the money to hire another nurse. In showing off, you risk not only making no gains but actually losing ground. Organizations offer some excellent marketing communication tools, which can add value to the physician relations effort and the overall referral relationships, including:

- Service line fact sheet
- Clinical outcomes data
- Trended data
- Research findings
- Clinical trials
- New CME topics
- New physician bios
- Current articles in clinical journals

**A Marketer's Guide to Physician Relations**

The most frequently used tools are a single-page sheet with an article or brief, a segment for data, and updates related to access, technology, or people. It's easily updated and offers a nice leave-behind for the representative and a good follow-up tool to set the stage for the next visit. Whenever possible, portray the data in graphs and charts; use statistics with meaning. Attractive packets with maps and a call-for-information number are very nice for patients—especially if you are a regional referral center. Give these to the office staff but not to the physician, who might not follow up.

For the most part, the office staff is interested in access, so consider a communication tool that makes it easy for the staff to find the resource it wants. Back in the day, it was a Rolodex card, a laminated sheet for the bulletin board, or a sticker on the fax machine. These methods aren't terribly impressive, and they're not guaranteed to get you business, but it will make it easier for the staff to find you. If you are charged with creating a communication piece for the practices, ask the physician relations representative to gather some field information for you. Although the representative can't conduct a full-blown survey, he or she can absolutely ask one or two questions to get an idea of what will work best. And remember, he or she is seeing the target physicians, who may give you a different reply than your loyal medical staff members.

**Teleservices.** The organization's ability to respond to a practice when it needs a consult, has an emergency to transfer, or wants to refer a patient to a specialist is foundational. Telemarketing is one tool that marketers really need to integrate, especially if they want to create a regional referral base. A well-run call center is an extension of marketing. It doesn't matter if the call center representatives report to the same person. What's important is synergy and connection to doing what is right to have those who want to send us business enjoy a positive and easy experience. If asked, your representatives will tell you that access is a critical difference-maker. I realize that this is not the sole responsibility of marketing but relies on operations and marketing working together to make this happen. The call center can be the nerve center for supporting calls from practices and facilitating connections to the specialists, access for transport, and appointment setting. Organizations go back and forth on whether to centralize or de-centralize the function, and there are naturally pros and cons to each.

East Texas (Tyler) Medical Center (ETMC) Regional Healthcare System has a centralized system to manage scheduling and the multiple needs of its regional referral sources. Centralizing really gives you the opportunity to take a marketing approach to intake and admissions; you are able to be more efficient and customer friendly, says Michael Thomas, VP of Strategic Planning and Marketing. The data you capture on a consistent basis will never be as good if you are decentralized, and marketing will not have that data in a way that can be used, tracked, measured, and analyzed. Across outpatient areas, when it has shifted the programs to a centralized scheduler, ETMC has consistently demonstrated an 18%–20% increase in volumes. Thomas admits that the standard routine is that if something goes wrong, it will be your fault, but having the facts to retrace the call and the details is possible only when you have a centralized center.

**A Marketer's Guide to Physician Relations**

Best-practice organizations spend significant time training call center staff to pay strong attention to customer service. Someone needs to own this and create organizational obligations for service because the physicians who are trying to send you business do not want to keep track of multiple phone numbers—they want one number, and they want consistent processes. Where the level of specificity is significant, there is a central call number, and physicians can contact individual departments as needed.

When organizations spend so much time, money, and effort on getting new business, a critical piece is access that is streamlined and welcoming. Here's a retail analogy: A superstore that wants to bring in all local business promotes itself regularly and frequently, explaining all the reasons it is superior to all the other stores. The customer, wowed by its qualities, comes to the store to try you out. Product in hand, the customer approaches the register. But then things break down. Rather than quickly and easily processing the transaction, the store makes everyone in line wait while the cashier calls for credit card authorization, opens the cash register drawer, and otherwise works hard to bring the store the money. This is a gross oversimplification, but if you want to grow business from new referral sources, you have to get serious about employing teleservices to support the growth.

Call centers are the best place to manage regional referral calls if they are engaged in the process, have the right staff, and train them well. Marketing must work with them to look beyond transactional obligations. There is significant opportunity to exemplify the brand in the personal style of inter-action and to cross-sell other programs and services when the opportunity arises. The other advantage of call center integration is improved reporting functions. Leverage the relationship to gather reports about those who are calling for appointments after the representative has visited. Give call center staff the names of "new prospects" so they flag the record and let you know if referrals have been generated. Use the call center team to let you know if there has been a troublesome referral so you can mend fences proactively. Some organizations rely heavily on data from the call center to prove ROI.

Large academic medical centers have significant challenges with managing the multiple, complex referral needs and the challenge of departmental autonomy. Often, there are opportunities to use the call center as the front door; then the call center is responsible for working through some of the internal channels to get patients to the right place, which is a far better approach than making a primary care office in the region try to do it.

Best-practice organizations use the combination of field research, market intelligence about how others do this, and streamlined systems of access that make it easy for physicians to send referrals their way. If it can't be ideal and there needs to be a bit of jerry-rigging behind the scenes, then manage these internal challenges so they do not become the referring physician's problem.

**Education.** If used well, one of the most powerful marketing tools we have is education. Those organizations that offer strong, proactive education essentially stake a claim as experts. Education includes the traditional CME offerings, which are excellent ways to provide value, create connections at a doctor-to doctor level, and demonstrate quality outcomes at your facility.

Beth Israel Deaconess Medical Center in Boston uses this tactic to highlight its clinical services and specialty physicians while also providing a valued service to their referring physicians. According to Elaine Monico, director of network development, a dedicated member of the team coordinates the specialists who are willing to be advocates through continuing medical education venues, liaison with community hospital CME coordinators for scheduling, and then communicate the schedule of events to the field staff who attend the sessions when possible to reinforce the referral development opportunity. Their goal is to conduct more than 100 sessions in 2007.

If there are CME programs targeted to a strategic service you are hoping to grow, use the representative to position the offering, extend the invitation, and encourage attendance. At times when a prospective new physician agrees to attend, the representative may even choose to meet the physician at the door and provide some introductions. The medium is education, but the experience is every bit as important.

Beyond CME venues, consider other ways to provide education. Many organizations have their specialists do educational updates within the region. These do not always need to include credit.

The use of education has been a strong element within the outreach model at Sunrise Health Systems in Las Vegas. "We traditionally received a fair number of transfers from rural hospitals to our tertiary center for cases they couldn't manage," says Director of Outreach Programs Sue Pietrafeso. "But then we had an epiphany that there is a real potential market here. So we would send out our specialists to do clinical education sessions. Additionally, we put together a dedicated team to accept telephone calls from referring facilities and streamline the process of getting patients transferred. With some structure, we were finally able to measure results and went from less than 100 cases per month to well over 320 cases per month."

A key to maximizing the impact of education is to have representatives follow up with the participants within two weeks after the event. That follow-up meeting becomes an opportunity to make certain that the participants learned something, to answer any questions, and to set the stage for the physician to refer patients who exhibit with the needs covered at the event to your facility.

**Public relations.** Some organizations have such strong public relations efforts in place that they are able to leverage this to position physicians and the physicians' expertise. We all recognize that physicians read the papers and watch TV, so the ability to position your specialists in the public eye can extend the recognition beyond consumer awareness. For those organizations that are working with regional providers, there is an excellent opportunity to develop stories for local publications that feature the local referring doctor and the specialist. A little free press goes miles in creating a credible relationship.

## Where does branding fit in all this?

"Many organizations have done an excellent job of implementing a branding strategy. Your brand is a valuable asset that must be conceived and managed with great acuity," says Margolis. "A strong brand envelops all communications. A hospital must communicate a clear, consistent, believable, straightforward image to all audiences, including physicians."

Physicians associate the brand not just with the message from the physician relations representative but their entire experience surrounding the organization. Often the messages and the implementation of the brand promise is not developed or implemented with the physician in mind. You must ensure that every interaction a physician has with your organization upholds the organization's brand positioning and delivers against its brand promise, says Margolis.

The actions of the CEO and other members of the senior management group most consistently communicate your brand to your physicians. Furthermore, if the employees understand the brand promise, their actions convey a strong message to the medical staff. Look at your brand through the eyes of the external physician. Step back and evaluate how you live the brand in daily physician interactions, both within the organization and as you work with them to admit their patients and as the representatives work to encourage new referrals.

## What are the must-haves?

With limited dollars and resources, there are tough choices to be made about the marketing that is allocated to the physician segment. Expensive brochures aren't the answer. Bread-and-butter marketing is the essential difference-maker. Integrate the physician relations strategies with the marketing plan, and look for ways to get more bang for the buck. Columbus Children's Hospital's Teach does zero-based planning each year—starting from scratch to look at what is in place and what should be in place. "There are no sacred cows in our shop," she says.

Anything and everything that can be done by marketing to support systems of access is the number-one thing. Beyond that, clinically oriented, up-to-date information is important. Although it has to look nice, it's content, not looks, that drives the acceptance for the physicians.

The physician relations program will function as a conduit for information, so there must be a sense of rapport and openness. If you are uncertain as to whether you need a printed physician guide, have the representatives ask a couple of questions of the target office staff when they are doing their visits. Always ask the question to make certain you are flexible in your approach to providing information. Some love everything online, while others still like a notebook or printed guide. The opportunity for physician relations, with a good relationship, is to take it to the next level. Offer to be active in communicating the brand at the physician level, and encourage marketing to share the promotional pieces with you. Share information with doctors before it hits the press. And encourage production of the type of materials that doctors will read and use.

# Pushing the envelope

Best-practice organizations realize that marketing to consumers and marketing to physicians are not mutually exclusive. The movement toward a consumer-driven market notwithstanding, many hospitals, health systems, and large specialty practices have revisited their allocation of marketing resources and, in some cases, are directing more resources toward physician marketing.

In fact, some programs have taken the next step in integrating physician relations and marketing by building a brand identity around their physician services in much the same way that organizations do for their consumer marketing. Initial efforts are most commonly directed toward branding and positioning the physician relations program in the marketplace. Some are working to extend the brand identity to all physician-related services and programs. Those taking this plunge often inventory their physician-related services throughout the organization in an attempt to organize these services into an integrated program. Not surprisingly, most organizations find a large number of physician-related services when they conduct the inventory. Common services include:

- Call center operations (physician-to-physician referral lines, nurse triage lines, and physician referral lines)

- Physician relations programs

- Physician retention programs

- Hospitalists (to support referring physicians)

- CME/educational programming

- Physician Web portals

- Newsletters and communication updates

- IT to support access to patient information by referring physicians (the complete medical record is ideal, but labs and radiology are helpful, too)

- Medical staff directories

- Physician recruitment

Clearly, not all of these programs will fall under the same reporting umbrella in most organizations. However, they can still be organized and delivered in a way that simplifies the life of the referring physician while enhancing the physician's ability to provide care for their patients.

The alternative to this comprehensive and integrated program approach is a fragmented array of services that appears confusing and disjointed to the referring physician. Once the behind-the-scenes implementation issues around integrating the services are resolved (and this is no small task, although the rewards are well worth the effort), then marketing can begin to aggressively

 **A Marketer's Guide to Physician Relations**

brand, position, and promote the program as a differentiating factor in the marketplace designed to meet physician needs. In all cases, key message points are developed and then communicated using traditional marketing tools (e.g., brochures, the Web, sales calls). These messages often revolve around items such as easy patient access, communication and follow-up with the referring physician, and access to the best clinical outcomes. In other cases, organizations have developed names, logos, and taglines for their programs in much the same way as their consumer marketing efforts. Although few do a great job of this, the expectations of referring physicians are relatively low. A simple but effective program can be successful in many markets, which provides additional time to build and refine the program.

Finally, as with any marketing efforts, measurement of outcomes and program impact is crucial. Common outcomes include name awareness of the program among the physician community; positive changes in physician satisfaction; and, ultimately, volume and/or revenue growth. There is tremendous advantage to having consistent messages reach physicians throughout the marketplace. Many leading marketers in the country are reaching out to better understand the physician and the breadth and depth of the tool kit that becomes a key area of differentiation. There is also a strong awareness of the key role that a physician relations effort imparts and how it fits into the total continuum.

## Operations, physician relations deliver the goods

Marketing and physician relations are logically seen as comparable services, but operations often seems like a far-distant universe. Old-timers remember healthcare when everything was supply-driven. There was little need to create a brand strategy, grow the referral base, or actively recruit new physicians. Enter intense competition and leaders who are actively engaged in growth strategies at every level. Marketing is doing its part, and physician relations is at the forefront of many leaders' plans for market-share increases.

Although the leaders are clearly embracing growth, many at the implementation level do not fully understand what it takes to grow business. The categories defined for the relationship with marketing are alive and well as we explore the clinical/physician relations efforts. Many clinical staffs are only mildly aware of the role of the physician liaison. Unless there has been a managed-care crisis or something similar, they are secure in their roles and rarely think about the competitive marketplace and business development strategy. It is simply outside their day-to-day concerns. Truth be told, many wish there were fewer patients, not more. Some see the physician relations team as a necessary evil. They do not always trust that the approach used is the right one, but they generally acknowledge that there is a need to have programs in place to grow interest.

Some organizations and departments, on the other hand, embrace the concept of growth. They are proactive, frequently led by an entrepreneurial doctor and a young and eager staff. I see more of this in the service lines or areas of the facility that are lower-revenue producers. Ironic, isn't it, that the service that is most accommodating and willing to work with the physician relations group is often the one that is least likely to be a strategic service? Maybe their leaders realize the value of new business to viability.

 **A Marketer's Guide to Physician Relations**

It's good to figure out where you are and then set a realistic expectation for where you need to be and when and how you'll get there. It is a must-have because physician relations will never reach its full potential without active clinical support. Successful relationship building and shifting of business is accomplished when the physician relations team learns to sell what can be delivered and when the clinical/operations team produces at a level equal and above expectations. But it does often mean that the physician relations team has to take the first step.

## Exceed expectations

The physician relations representative is obligated to position what can be delivered. When the service underdelivers, the organization doesn't yield real results. It's a short-term win for the representative. Best-practice organizations create a shared approach that works and yields results. Working with the clinical team, the messages must describe the services that are provided. When creating the messages, the physician relations team will push for the maximum offerings and often needs to work hard to determine what is different.

There must also be a clear understanding of who does what in the process—not to lay all the detail on the prospective practice but to understand where the process may break down. The physician relations team also needs to understand the types of patients that qualify for the services and from whom they would generally be referred. For example, are these patients that would already be in the care of a cardiologist, or would a family physician likely refer them into the facility? When can the patients get in, and how long does it take before the patient/referring physician gets a diagnosis? Excessive wait times are often not seen as excessive at all by the internal staff, so it is important to have the average and then share the correct information. In the event that it really is excessive, then you have the obligation to position those services that are perceived as valuable and market-test the time expectations. It is good to understand what is inpatient, what is outpatient, and what is clinic only. As the representative works with the practice, where the service is delivered can potentially be a key area of service differentiation from competitors.

### Why is there strong market interest in the service?

This is really the sizzle part of the message, the ability to position your service offering at a different level than the competition (without giving the competition any floor time). In my experience, this is not information that is readily thought about by the operational team, so the physician relations team or marketing staff must gather this detail and then confirm it with the clinical leaders. Susan Milford at Centegra Health has used her marketing staff to orchestrate the message management, and it has proven very effective. They are able to extract the right detail for their marketing communication strategy and then support the physician relations effort with consistent message management.

## The specialist's office

Although most of our focus is at the organization level, the ability to deliver the product starts with the referring physician's entry into the system via a

**A Marketer's Guide to Physician Relations**

practice. Although academic environments have their faculty physicians in this role, there are some who have employed physician specialists, and many facilities rely on private practices to be their access point into the system. Some organizations have worked hard to streamline access and support the appointment-setting process at the clinic level in hopes of providing excellent customer service.

ETMC has a fairly innovative approach to this and one that has made a significant impact. To support its regional clinics with referrals, it has stationed a referral coordinator in the key offices. Although this might seem like a cost-prohibitive idea, ETMC has found it to be a significant cost benefit. The service is excellent, referrals stay within the system, and the patient care is streamlined because the paperwork and processes are complete.

Consider these proactive approaches to ensure that the referring physician has success with getting practice appointments:

- Centralize scheduling services.

- Work with office staff or provide customer service and education programs for the receptionists. This is especially appropriate for your strategic service areas.

- Keep objective detail about what works well and what does not. If you need to go back to the practice, you must have objective data.

- Create a backdoor service recovery strategy, similar to the one Columbus Children's Hospital offers. Ask the practices to give you one more chance before they take the business elsewhere.

- When you are focused on promotion of a service area, determine the access approach, issues, and wait times. Know the baseline before you start. If there are significant barriers, sit down with the practice administrator or the lead physician to develop a solution.

- Meet with the specialists who will be the benefactors of the growth strategy. Create an agenda and openly discuss your needs and expectations, but also take care to learn their needs and expectations. This is your chance to ask the tough questions, such as how the specialist wants the organization to communicate with him or her. This gives the specialist a chance to think it through, and you can then make note of his or her management structure and style.

## The role of the representative in service delivery

While best-practice organizations focus on the external-relationship strategy, they also understand the pivotal role representatives play in making sure the products and services are correctly represented and delivered at the level expected. For the physician relations representative, there are three obligations that relate to service delivery:

1. To properly position the products and services

 **A Marketer's Guide to Physician Relations**

2. To gather objective details about what went wrong when the service was not delivered as promised

3. To represent the team and all its members in the most positive light

Representatives sometimes get caught up in their conversations with prospective referring physicians and make promises beyond what the organization can deliver. Generally, it is an innocent slip on the part of an overenthusiastic salesperson bent on growing referrals. Instead of saying, "We may be able to do that," he or she says "We'll always be able to do that." In healthcare, it drives the operations team absolutely nuts. As a group of individuals who like process—and do not like it when people expect more than they were prepared to offer—this can cause some bad vibes between the parties. The best solution is to sell to the minimum expectations that can be consistently offered. Here's how it works:

- **Learn through questions.** When representatives are learning about a new service or product, they should ask lots of detailed questions to understand clearly the product's scope and availability. For example, they might ask whether the physician must order certain tests before his or her patient would be seen for a certain procedure—and any other questions that the referring physician would ask.

- **Get promises for sales differentiators.** Representatives should ask the clincher question—what can they promise the physician? For example, the representative might say, "I heard you say that often the wait time is only a day or two. That tells me sometimes it may be later. Can I promise with 100% certainty that patients are always seen within a week? What is the absolute always, knowing we often beat that?"

- **Create your messages.** The next step is for the representatives to create messages that focus on the minimum expectations that will be met 100% of the time. Operations can help develop the key messages, particularly in the areas of patient benefits and outcomes. Taking the time to think about the messages will give you more confidence in your tone and less likelihood of overpromising.

- **Get it in writing.** Summarize these "agreements" in a simple summary sheet, and provide them to the service line leader for his or her files. The representatives sell the service at this level, and when the organization exceeds expectations, so much the better. It's sort of like the game show "The Price is Right." If you underbid, even by a lot, you're in the game. But if you are just $1 over, you're out of the game. In physician relations, if you underpromise and overdeliver, you're still in the game. Overpromise and underperform? Game over.

- **Build your case if minimum doesn't cut it.** It's not possible to always be the most, best, quickest, and cheapest. But there are times when the minimum will just not create any leverage for you to grow the business. If the minimum level of service negotiated in this process isn't acceptable to create interest, document physicians' responses in the field. With solid documentation about their expectations and market intelligence

**A Marketer's Guide to Physician Relations**

about what competing facilities are offering, meet with service line leadership. For example, if your facility says it can consistently schedule patients for routine stress tests two months out and the competitor routinely schedules patients within two days, your consistency is useless and will never get tested or tried.

- **Gather objective details when the service is not delivered as promised.** What if the clinical team agrees to schedule MRIs within seven days and then does not meet this promise on a consistent basis? First and foremost, follow up with service line leaders and get senior leadership involved. It's far too much work to not have both parties live up to their obligations. Although the physician relations team can take the first step and be proactive, there must be a commitment to service delivery on both sides.

## Engaging clinical staff in the field

One of the themes of this chapter is involvement. As we look at what relationship needs must be met to grow market share, we turn to the internal partners to help us fulfill those needs. Best-practice organizations actively work to include their department heads and clinical service leads whenever a prospective physician needs more information or when there is an opportunity to differentiate the organization through a higher-caliber staff. This works best when the representative has a face-to-face meeting with the prospective physician to position the service and the individual. At the next meeting, the representative brings along the internal expert for a clinically based dialogue.

At the end, the representative closes—either scheduling a return visit or asking for the referral opportunity, depending on the discussion. Success depends on the following:

**The right clinical expert.** It must be someone who has strong communication skills and understands the role is to help position the service so you can get new business. He or she must also have strong knowledge. Because this person is being positioned as the internal expert, he or she must have lots of depth and breadth of detail.

**An expert who doesn't take over.** The clinical expert must understand dialogue and the role of the representative. This is an area where best-practice programs invest dollars for training to teach clinicians the dynamics of the relationship sales call.

**The ability to qualify the opportunity.** It is the role of the representative to qualify the prospective physician. Based on the learnings, the specific needs are shared with the clinician so he or she can develop talking points that are relevant to the prospective physician in advance of the discussion.

**A clear path for closure, actions, and next steps.** It is the representative's job to close the meeting. This might mean securing a return visit that will focus on gaining referral commitment, getting the physician's commitment to more referral business, or another step toward referral commitment, such as a CME opportunity, physician visit, or a staff tour of the campus. All these closes are fine—the point is that the clinical person should be confident that the representative will take care of this.

# Problems in paradise

Best-practice organizations know that not everyone will deliver exemplary service at your facility every time. They create management tools to deal with physician complaints, not unlike the approach they use to deal with patient complaints. If the program goal is to keep their representatives focused on growth, they must have a method for dealing with the issues. Otherwise, the issues will bury the representative. Although there are some variations in process and approach, these elements are consistent in the best ones:

**An internal champion is critical to success.** Effective issue-resolution processes start with someone who is committed to recognizing that physician satisfaction with services is vital to success. This can be a COO, a division chief, a physician with oversight for quality, or the chief medical officer. Whoever it is, he or she must have clout within your organization and have the ability to get the attention of those accountable for the fix.

The program champion often becomes the mouthpiece for the program. He or she pushes the issue agenda at leadership meetings, manages outliers who do not respond to problems within the allotted time, rolls out the top issues, and works with the right internal experts to create long-term solutions.

The champion's role cannot be underestimated. Issue resolution is one of those programs that needs almost constant attention. A passionate leader makes certain that the organization is working to gain new business because of exemplary level of caregiving and follow-through that exceeds expectations.

**The physician relations representatives must gather accurate, objective details.** Today's representative understands that the nature of the role is not to go looking for problems. But when they do occur, he or she must manage them. The starting point is always to gather objective detail. My approach is to ask the physician whether I can work with the office manager or his/her nurse to garner specific detail. This has proven to be a good technique because the doctor usually does not have all the facts. Physicians are relieved to pass it on, and our conversation can then progress to other topics of interest. If the nurse does not have enough detail to pass on, I do let the doctor know and alert the staff to call me personally so I can document the details if it should occur again.

One of the greatest frustrations for operations staff is when a representative comes to the staff with absolutes. We "never" do something, or we "always" fail to do something else. Remind representatives that if they cannot provide details and evidence to back up complaints, they won't be able to take the fix back to the physician. To assist with this process, the physician relations team benefits from a standard issue documentation sheet. It is always best if the operations team has created the sheet; make sure it's one sheet that can be used hospitalwide—not a sheet for each department. It will detail the patient detail, date of occurrence, what the practice expected to occur, and the contact person for follow-up. It needs to have enough detail to track down the issue but should not require a full history.

**Timelines and accountabilities are critical.** Everyone is too busy; we live for deadlines, and most of us work just one step ahead of them. Best-practice organizations have delineated deadlines for responding to issues and clear channels for who communicates and how it is documented.

In general, most programs state that the practice will have a reply within 48 hours. Although the problem has not always been solved in that time, there can be a status report. There is often internal pushback from those who, at the 48-hour mark, say there is nothing to report. This is not a good approach. Push the operations people to offer a reply regardless of the final answer. Physicians will appreciate knowing that someone heard them and is working to find a solution.

The best programs have specific ownership obligations. Accountability is about making certain that the individuals who lead the problem area own the solution. The department heads are often held responsible for making the initial call and ensuring a solution and/or an explanation. The chairs or department leaders are not always the ones who fix the problem, but they are always accountable.

**Problems are best managed by those who have oversight for the departments and services in which they occurred.** Someone needs to own the problem, and the best owner is the individual who can actually do something about it.

Job performance evaluations need to be tied to a person's ability to effect the change or to communicate why it cannot be fixed and whether steps are being taken to explore future solutions.

Again, this is where the program champion plays a significant role. Like the implementation of so many programs, almost everyone plays by the rules and does his or her best to respond. Then there's that one department that chooses to do its own thing. There must be consistent implementation, and the program champion needs to be empowered to make certain everyone abides by the policies or be disciplined. The greatest challenges arise when there are multidepartmental breakdowns. And there's a reason why they have been ignored—it's because there is no easy solution. The role of the physician relations team is to track and measure so there is a strong and compelling need to create the solution.

**Tracking tools are essential.** To manage issue resolution effectively, there are several touchpoints where details must be tracked to determine the individual issue, response, and impact and to roll up the organization's issues and better understand the consistency with which an issue may be occurring and the type of business that is lost because of it.

Some organizations use patient complaint software, whereas others use the tracking tools from their physician database software. Any system purchased for this purpose must be carefully tested to determine ease of use. Most need some customization, and they all need some support in the reporting.

The most effective issue resolution reporting is an element within the leadership reports that lists the number of issues by category, what is being done, and whether there is potential to change referral relations for this dollar amount. Use data rather than lots of stories, although sometimes it is the story that drives the momentum. For example, point out that 62% of physicians are unhappy with OR scheduling or that 7% wanted quicker turnaround on lab tests. With this type of detail, it is clear that the OR scheduling is not just one or two whiney physicians.

Remember that this is the very group of doctors that we want to send us more business. Managing issues is often expanded to a hospitalwide process and tracking approach. With the successful management and resolution of issues that are demonstrated through sales, organizations become very interested in expanding the methodology to manage issues that are learned by other leaders or stakeholders. Issues are likely to be less frequent among splitters and nonusers.

Hospitals that have retention programs in place with either leaders or liaisons working to maintain those referrals are more likely to share concerns. The process and approach for tracking and measuring is very effective for this group as well. The only difference is that sometimes with strong retention programs, the liaison is much more actively involved in communicating the solution to the physician.

With sales programs, the decision is often made to have the operations staff "own the solution" and share the solution directly with the physician and office and then send a note of resolution off to the staff. Don't overengineer this. Keep communications simple. To be effective, everyone involved must understand the process for success. Because of the number of people involved and the nature of the attention, it is easy to make this more extravagant than it needs to be. Resist that temptation.

Listen carefully, respond appropriately, track the challenges and the "cure rate," and use this to leverage communication. If you are just developing your model, first test it with the physician relations process and then expand the model to other entry points within the organization.

## Best-practice models

There are many variations of the basic physician complaint resolution model detailed here. The following model uses a six-step process to respond to physician concerns:

**Step 1: Intake.** The physician relations representative collects and documents details about the issue.

**Step 2: Triage.** The issue is assigned to the appropriate individual(s) and/or department for review and resolution, and the physician is notified of the process in a timely fashion.

Two approaches are used to triage and assign the issue to the appropriate individuals or department in the organization. The first is a "centralized"

**A Marketer's Guide to Physician Relations**

approach, in which the sales staff directs the issue to an individual who then assigns a responsible party. The second is a "direct" approach, in which the sales staff seeks out the appropriate individual or group in the organization and makes the assignment on its own. With the first approach, the sales staff generally hands over the issue to a member of the senior leadership team (e.g., CEO, COO, chief medical officer, or chief nursing officer), and this individual makes the appropriate assignment. With the second approach, the sales staff solicits assistance from the individual(s) or department in the organization best situated to respond to the issue. Most organizations have a standing requirement that the physician registering the complaint is contacted within 48 hours.

**Step 3: Processing.** During this stage, the issue is reviewed, and opportunities to improve processes are assessed. The length of time in this stage depends on the complexity of the issue. (Some issues are resolved in hours, while others may take weeks.)

**Step 4: Status updates.** The physician and sales staff are updated regarding issue status, new developments, etc. There are two schools of thought on the update process. Most of the best-practice models have the clinical and operational staff accountable for timely communication with the physician and sales staff regarding issue status and updates. Having clinical and operational staff responsible increases the likelihood of timely resolution while removing this time burden from sales. There are some organizations that use the representative to find and communicate the solution to the physician. This is seen more often when their territory includes both growth and retention.

**Step 5: Closure.** The issue is closed, and the final outcome is communicated to the physician and sales staff.

**Step 6: Tracking and reporting.** Issues are tracked throughout the entire process, and various reports are produced for the sales staff and senior leadership.

## Using feedback to improve quality and outcomes

One of the most impressive and most rewarding aspects of this approach to issue resolution is that complaints are not front and center, but when they occur, there is an ability to communicate them in a proactive way and to get solutions. Often it is much more than a doctor who has a beef—there are also quality and safety challenges that can cost the organization dearly when not well managed. Take the time to create tools and techniques to work with the operations team and enhance the integration. There is no better collaborative team.

# A physician-centric culture

Once your physician relations representatives (backed by all the best practices described in the book so far) convince their target physicians to send new business to the hospital, what happens next? The hospital must welcome the physicians and allow them to practice medicine in the style they desire. Best-practice organizations understand this and create service recovery mechanisms to ensure that business is delivered as promised. The best physician relations representatives also know that there is never value in making promises that the organization can't keep.

Many of the best practices I've described so far are possible for the physician relations team to initiate, support, and implement. For me, these best practices are easier to talk about and share tips and techniques for because of the several ways they can be implemented. They have attributes that are designed to engage the prospective referral source and to encourage him or her to refer new business to the organization. But the last two best-practice areas discussed in the book are the ones that really push programs to better performance.

In this chapter, I'll discuss creating a physician-centric culture, which is all about the environment within the healthcare organization. This is an area where the representative has limited impact. But it's important when you're trying to build long-term satisfaction, create more meaningful relationships, and make the referring physician feel valued.

## Physician-focused customer service

In the past 7–10 years, there has been an explosion of interest in customer service. It has put patient satisfaction and employee relationships front and center. To enhance the physician experience, start by assessing the current relationship that your organization has with its medical staff, how it got to be this way, and what must be done to improve it. It's not enough to replicate patient or employee satisfaction tools. The physician's relationship, knowledge, issues, options, and expectations are much different than consumers'. Physicians are also in a very different place in terms of their own business satisfaction. It is critically important that we step back and assess the current environment for them and with them and then craft the right cultural approach.

Physician-centric customer service is almost exclusively out of the hands of the physician relations team. So why is it a best practice for physician relations? Because for the physician relations team to be effective, it must be able to deliver a desirable service, with all that entails. The goal is to get repeat business from referring physicians and for them to become more committed to your organization. You can have an outstanding physician

**A Marketer's Guide to Physician Relations**

relations program, but if the physician believes that the representative is the only one in the organization who wants the physician to refer, then all the effort is wasted.

Focus on physicians is a best practice because the representative's role is to earn the referral and the organization's role is to ensure that the physician feels as though the decision to refer to your organization was the right one. The organization must assure the physician of his wisdom in changing referral locations by creating the right environment.

## What you need to begin

For most organizations, the thought of a full-fledged overhaul of their customer service approach for physicians is overwhelming. Most aren't willing to take it on unless there is a crisis in the ranks or things have gone so well with their service initiatives that it would add value. The tendency is to minimize relationship challenges, especially since there are so many other issues facing today's leadership teams.

If you believe that physician customer service deserves more attention, the best approach is to maximize the positives from a relationship-building role and then provide objective documentation for the areas that you believe need improvement. For example, if the chief operating officer (COO) does an exceptional job of responding to physician needs, ask him or her to meet with prospective physicians.

For the relationship to move forward, the representative must find a way to position what is positive. And rather than be frustrated by the lack of service from some areas, document the specifics, and include them in the regular report. Often this documentation will result in the leadership taking action to enhance communication and responsiveness. That is the first step in a cultural change. There are several small steps that can build on one another, having a very positive impact. Not surprisingly, the first of these involves the organization's leaders.

## Leaders who listen

With so many different voices in the business environment—not to mention the number of hidden messages and political agendas—it's hard to really listen these days. Leaders have multiple constituents, each of whom wants something from them. This is further complicated by the fact that physicians are not always the best at explaining what they feel, what they need, or how serious the issue is. Leaders who listen well have the following attributes:

- They make corrections based on "little things" that are said

- They ask questions to hear more fully, to gather background, and to understand what the physician would suggest as an alternative

- They give both positive and negative feedback to staff

- They demonstrate active listening for their staff

© 2007 HCPRO, INC.    **A Marketer's Guide to Physician Relations**

We all know leaders who have a wonderful knack for cutting through the clutter and really connecting with a member of the medical staff. When you analyze their behavior, the essence of what happens is that they listen. Their actions are not assumptive. They heard what the doctor wants and needs. These leaders create a welcoming environment. Their style and approach is evident in their relationship building. Some say they just simply don't have time to practice this approach and listen to every doctor who wants to bend their ear. In reality, listening and responding in the right way the first time saves significant time, energy, and money. And that the relationship goodwill is hard to even measure.

"Open communication with physician partners characterizes physician-focused organizations," says Burl Stamp, president and founder of Stamp & Chase, Inc., in St. Louis. Leadership listens to physicians' ideas on major issues that affect their practices and the operation of the hospital. Leadership also actively shares rationale for decisions so that physicians understand the background and key considerations, even if they do not agree with the final decision.

There's an easy way to gather physicians' insights and see where your organization needs to improve. Working with leadership, the physician relations representative can craft a couple of questions to gain the physician's perspectives on responsiveness. After all, responsiveness is a visible sign of listening. The feedback will be from those physicians who have growth potential, not those who are currently fairly loyal if you use the target groups, so you may want to have the internal retention experts ask the same questions and then compare the pools as you craft your plan. Consider asking the following questions:

- When you have a suggestion for new technology, who do you find is the best person to share that information with?

- What is your desired turnaround time after you share a concern with a member of the hospital leadership? Does this happen?

- How do the hospital leaders currently gather information on the needs of the medical staff? How effective is this?

## A proactive strategy

Many of the best-practice organizations have a robust and focused retention approach. They recognize that the competition would love to lure away physicians who actively admit, so they have created a formal methodology for enhancing loyalty, involvement, and satisfaction. This is not unlike the growth strategy in its approach: regular visits, dialogue in the physician's office or the hospital, or involvement strategies for those who are clinic-based and rely on hospitalists. This can include both social and educational events. These leaders often use quality and outcomes at the center of their messages and work to let doctors know that they understand the challenges they face. None of this is easy, but it makes a tremendous difference in long-term relationship building and in creating the right culture within. It obviously has an impact on those physicians who are directly touched by the proactive retention, but it also changes the overall feel of the entire medical staff. Niceness breeds niceness.

The retention model can take many different forms. The most important aspect is that there is consistency, so the same person is connecting with the retention physician on a regular (at least quarterly) basis. As well, the connections are proactive and designed to share messages and learn perceptions. The nature of these visits is that there will often be more concerns shared. After all, these doctors are invested enough in your facility to complain. In a culture that welcomes physicians, there is a clearly defined mechanism for solving issues and reporting the solution back to the physician.

## An open spirit

Some leadership teams say that they can't acquiesce to the doctors' every whim. Much of what they want is not legal, and often there is no good business logic to back up their requests. Welcoming environments don't say "yes" to every physician every time. But they do other things. They have an open-door policy, for example. They proactively learn the needs of their constituents. They have a consistent communication style and approach. They tell the physician what they will do with a request and then they do just that. Best practices encourage new ideas by responding in a positive light whenever they can, and they are always consistent in providing rationale and details when they have to say no to a request.

## Physician representation

At best-practice organizations, physicians' needs are clearly represented. This, of course, means that they have board representation, but it also means that the hospital has a large pool of physicians to tap for ideas and suggestions. This is true for policy and departmental issues as well as overall strategic issues. Find regular ways to involve doctors in the right level of decision-making at the hospital. It is hard to bash decisions when you were part of making them. When you must say no to physicians, make sure that they hear it first and that it is told to them with the right level of leadership and the rationale. Cultures that work to gain and maintain the respect of their medical staff ensure that the leadership team, often the CEO, finds the physician and talks directly to him or her.

Those organizations that are further along with this cultural recognition realize that physicians will make decisions that will ensure their long-term financial viability and that do not have a negative impact on the care they give to their patients. In some organizations, there are still individuals who choose to paint physicians as bad people because they make financially beneficial decisions. Granted, there are some doctors who fit in this category, but often their business needs are just that—business, not personal.

There are times when the organization cannot create a win-win situation. This is evident when competing groups both want their needs met or they have issues with a payer who is going to cause significant turmoil, yet it is unavoidable. Those organizations that fostered a good relationships before this are certainly able to weather the challenges with more opportunity to rebuild.

Doug Crabtree, CEO of Eastern Idaho (Idaho Falls) Regional Medical Center, went through a significant upheaval as a small group of physicians built a separate hospital in their community. The hospitals opted to take a stand, and the splits and turmoil in the market were overwhelming. But with a recognition

**A Marketer's Guide to Physician Relations**

that no one would win if the battle continued, the hospital decided to move forward, accept the change, and rebuild those relationships. In the end, the balance happens with the little things. "Physicians rightfully seek hospital partners that truly 'walk the talk,' not just espouse a physician focus in public forums and official publications," says Stamp.

Dave Flicek, senior vice president (VP) of clinic operations at Avera McKennan in Sioux Falls, SD, agrees. "A doctor once told me, 'It comes down to parking tickets, Dave. If I'm always getting a parking ticket when I park downtown, pretty soon the mall looks pretty good,' " he says. "It's the little hassle factors that just turn people bitter. So our goal is to try and make those little hassle factors nonexistent as much as possible."

## Creative business opportunities

Many organizations are working to align business strategies, be it with partnerships, employment either full time or for a hospital-based function, or other creative affiliations. Physician-focused organizations explore the possibilities, share what they can or cannot do, and find forthright messages to communicate.

The figure on the next page describes the role of physician relations within the greater context of the relationship strategy. Although there are business relationships that require different structures and often provide for the alignment of financial interests, much of this is done by business development.

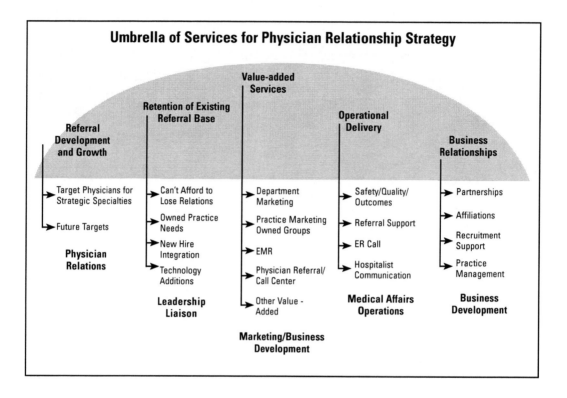

**Umbrella of Services for Physician Relationship Strategy**

There are certainly a large number of organizations that are focused on affiliation agreements and big-picture options for shoring up the business relationship. These include:

- Employment options
- Recruitment support
- Joint-venture relationships
- Shared equity in real estate
- Payment for duties, such as directorships, program development, etc.
- Call pay

 **A Marketer's Guide to Physician Relations**

The call-pay issue is a sensitive topic. In some markets, the specialists demand payment for their coverage. It is certainly not an area that most leaders are eager to explore, and most are exploring options and trying to work closely with physician leaders to manage this.

Certainly the revenue-sharing options are critical, but there are ways that organizations work to demonstrate creative interest in having and keeping their referrals. While there is huge growth in this area, others continue to provide more business and management support with a physician-focused orientation.

Avera McKennan made a conscious decision to build a site-based model for physician employment with a decentralized management approach. "One big decision we had to make was to keep the billing local," says Flicek. "And that was against all of the hospital concepts about practice management. But with the physicians paid based on each patient they see, the billing slips are like paychecks. And if you ship that 200 miles away, there is concern that it is not being done right. So our philosophy is to give them control over what they can control. It's just like private practice—you worry about the accounts receivable and the charges, and we will take off your backs the contracts, malpractice costs, etc. We help weather the storm rather than taking things over."

The economics are another critical element, although they do not stand alone. You can buy friends (or physicians) short term, but the long-term strategy must also align with communication. They need to feel part of the organization; they need support, guidance, and trust as well. In a 2005 HealthCare Advisory Board Report, 74% of those surveyed indicated a need for assistance in business and management performance of their clinic. So even if your board members or leaders are not yet ready to change their practice model, there may be some other value-added options that can buy time and create goodwill in the short run.

With its academic partners, Beth Israel Deaconess Medical Center in Boston has created a collaborative outreach effort within its network-development function. Director of Network Development Elaine Monico describes the program. "We have built partnerships with community organizations to help them establish a higher level of clinical offering and provide brand image to support the local hospital and its ability to be competitive. We will supply hospitalists, surgical-service expertise, clinical trials for their cancer patients, and help them advance into cardiac angioplasty. All of this is through the physicians both at our organization and the local hospital. Then we, as management, just put the details around what the physicians determine is needed to augment local services and advance clinical care," she says.

Organizations explore creative business models for two reasons. Some are interested only in the dollars and the short-term gains of "doing the deal." Those are clearly not the ones that we call out as best practices in creating a physician-centric environment. At the end of the day, it is much more about the spirit in which these business options are offered. The ones that fall into the best-practice category recognize this as one element of a multipronged plan, and while, yes, the financial viability is a pivotal part of the decision process, a relationship strategy is seen as essential for the long term.

**A Marketer's Guide to Physician Relations**

# What do physicians want?

We've had lots of discussion about what organizations should provide and how they should provide it. It begs the questions, "What is it that the physicians really want?" and "What attributes would make the organization be the ultimate welcoming environment for physicians?" If only there was some magic formula that would explain how to satisfy every doctor. Those of us who have raised kids know that what you do with one child may or may not work with the next. The greatest challenge we face here is assuming we know what physicians want without asking, learning, listening, and offering some options. That said, there are some fundamentals we must provide, including:

**Quality care.** A safe environment for his or her patients is a basic requirement for every physician. Clinical outcomes are at the heart of this, so regular involvement and reporting of outcomes, issues, process improvement, and physician involvement are key. Physicians also evaluate safety based on their perceptions of staffing, especially nurses. There is always a cry for more nurses, but, beyond that, they are looking for consistency in the nursing ranks. And for those specialists who are at the hospital regularly, they like to see the leaders on the floors and in the clinical areas observing and supporting the clinical-care issues.

**Ease of access.** All doctors want easy access—for admitting patients, performing procedures, and gaining information. If you are uncertain how you are performing in this regard, perform mystery shopping to learn about wait times, service approach, and the challenges a practice faces when it wants to get patients scheduled. Beyond scheduling just one test, see how it works when you need to have a series of tests scheduled. If you want to grow surgical cases, physician relations representatives can gather the market expectations for you as part of the visit. Remember, if you are going to grow the business, you must be consistently at or above the desired access time.

**Excellent staff.** Physicians want to practice at a location that attracts other first-rate clinical staff and especially other top-notch physicians. Physicians will tell you that what makes their hospital a quality place is the medical staff's level of expertise. They like to be surrounded by others who are well thought of in the medical community.

**Credit where credit is due.** Physicians love visible signs that you recognize their contributions and their challenges. This certainly starts with understanding the world of medical practice and the challenges physicians face with finances, malpractice, staffing, and the hassle factors of too much paperwork and declining reimbursement. Focused organizations include physician leadership in developing the organization's long-term strategy.

Physician membership on formal strategic planning committees convened by the hospital is, of course, essential. But physician involvement must go beyond officially sanctioned committees. Important strategic decisions often happen outside the structured planning process, and the physician perspective must be reflected in this continual assessment and adjustment of the strategy. But it goes further. It is also about valuing their perspective on the changing world of medicine and being actively involved in those meetings that have a direct impact.

**A Marketer's Guide to Physician Relations**

Best-practice organizations realize that if physicians are not making the time to be involved with their efforts, it is because there is limited value for the physician.

## Measuring success

An institution that is truly physician-focused will reap the rewards in measurable business success. But watching these measures alone is not sufficient to gauge emerging trends and monitor physician mind-set toward the organization. The most effective institutions know exactly where they stand with their medical staffs because they consistently measure attitudes and actions in both qualitative and quantitative ways. At a basic level, hospitals must measure and monitor exactly where admissions and referrals are coming from. This includes the primary care referrals as we discussed early on, in addition to knowing which specialist actually admits them.

The other quantitative measure hospitals must assess on a regular basis is overall physician attitudes and practice patterns. A structured physician satisfaction tool administered by a third-party organization is the most effective way to attain this information across medical staff specialties and within defined geographic practice areas. This type of global survey should be fielded at least every two years—more frequently in more turbulent, markets.

Qualitative research is an essential complement to quantitative information. A hospital's physician services team provides the first line of defense in this area—if the information and knowledge obtained is effectively captured and shared with key decision-makers and operations leaders throughout the hospital. Too often, great sales reports with valuable insights and information are closely held within the physician services department when they could be most beneficial to operations executives and managers. If sales reports are used primarily as a way to document the time and work of physician representatives, the organization misses their real value. Those who do it best are always looking to improve on what is working. Stagnancy is never an option in the quest to be a best practice!

**A Marketer's Guide to Physician Relations**

# Ability to differentiate

No matter what you call it, a physician relations program is, at its heart, a sales effort. Best-practice organizations understand that it's not what the programs have to offer physicians that's important. Rather, it is what their customers need and want that matters. Best-practice organizations know how to package and position the services that are of interest to prospective referring physicians. For many organizations, however, there is often rabid internal interest in pushing a product without taking the time to explore whether there is interest, capacity, and enough of the right type of buyers in the market to make it viable.

## So many sales pitches, so little time

Sometimes physician relations representatives feel like just another messenger in a sea of representatives all saying the same thing: "Try me! Try me! Here I am!" Market clutter is a huge problem. And clamoring to get the physician's attention will not help you cut through it. It's great if your organization can find a way to create an edge. The challenge is to find a way to make an impact and develop your position with everyone else trying to do the same. Those who will be successful in the end are the ones who listen to what physicians need and then work with the internal stakeholders to craft the right message.

There is infinitely more to this than a smooth-tongued message. It starts with the ability to deliver something of interest and ends with consistency. If we are going to differentiate what we offer, we must be able to feel confident that the benefits we describe are delivered every time.

For physician relations, it also means we must minimize the risk—real or perceived—associated with a referral change. Often physicians stay with their current referral patterns not because they know them to be best but because they know them and they know exactly what they will get—good, bad, or indifferent. We also need to ensure that the message is delivered in a way that is logical so the physician thinks that it is, in part, his or her own idea to shift business.

The obligation to create a unique position is not understood by many internal leaders, who are banking on the sales effort alone to grow business. When you work inside the organization, your passion for the services, the people, and the processes blinds you to the multiple other organizations that are offering similar services. It's what we love about our people. But it doesn't make someone who has "never been one of us" feel compelled to do business with us.

The ability to differentiate is the culmination of many of the other best-practice efforts, but it's also more. It's knowing how to take what you have and what the market will let you be and package it in a way that puts you top of mind as a provider that deserves to earn new business. It is strategic and requires focus. It also demands that you clearly understand what the competition has to offer.

## How capable staffs help

Capable staffs are critical to differentiation for two reasons. They are able to stay on message and clearly articulate the key elements of differentiation. Capable staffs also manage the internal pleas to peddle multiple messages and resist the misguided notion that if the representative just tells the doctors all that the organization has to offer, then the physicians will send more referrals.

The essence of how you differentiate comes from service delivery. How you work with the internal operational team creates a level of service or technology that stands out. And the ability to continue to earn the new business and to allow the physician to feel valued, if done well, gives you the opportunity to leverage the position you have earned. The result is that physicians feel a level of confidence in their choice for patient care. But, is that enough to really know that you have the best program? No. Although these best practices are synergistic, there is more to having a clearly differentiated program than that.

Many programs are finding ways to differentiate themselves through strategy, staffing, and operational excellence. It is the next level of differentiation that really pushes us all.

# Make promises that matter

Business professionals know that it is important to select accessories that match their attire. Even those who do not consider themselves mall moguls are aware that if you have on black slacks, you ought to wear black shoes. Yet, as we sometimes put our message accessories together, we find ourselves in those sleek black slacks and some Birkenstock sandals. Each is lovely, each has its place, but the black slacks person should not try to do the Birkenstock thing.

In the same way, be careful about the service position that you select to differentiate your program, especially with that group of physicians that is not giving you as much business as you'd like. The service position must match who you really are as an organization. If you are an academic medical center, the message of being flexible and offering easy access at the front end may not make sense. Although you may have made great improvements in these areas, it's not what you're known for, nor is it the reason that physicians refer their patients to you. This is a back-end service requirement; it is not the key to differentiating your service capabilities.

Even if physicians have in the past complained about your access system, and even if you have made vast improvements to it, access is valuable only if the physicians want to do business with you first. The message strategy, then, is to differentiate your academic expertise, perhaps through breadth of specialties and clinical sophistication. Improved access is an additional value—no physician will automatically change a referral pattern because

**A Marketer's Guide to Physician Relations**

there are fewer hoops to jump through for access. The reason physicians seek
you out as an academic medical center is your outstanding clinical capability.
If this was not the case, and access could stand alone, why would everyone
not be in the suburbs for care? Donna Teach, vice president (VP) of marketing
and public relations at Nationwide Children's Hospital in Columbus, OH,
calls this getting her organization into the consideration set. "You've got to
be in a physician's referring set for them to even consider referring to you,"
she says. "That's where the reputational marketing, program benefits, and
program attributes make them consider you among one of the places they
would refer to."

Know your differentiators, the value-added messages, and the support
messages for your organization. Recognize what can be a compelling reason
to risk change, and that becomes central to shifting business.

## Deliver on promises consistently

Make sure that you can actually demonstrate what you are differentiating.
Empty promises are so damaging to a relationship with a physician. The world
of the physician is not about "almost right." Physicians are scientists who like
things in terms of black and white, and if we tell them we do something, they
expect that we will. Physicians want us to be straight with them and tell them
what we can and cannot do. This holds true for our differentiated message
and for our value-added messages. Physicians will quickly see through false
promises, and they will not be back. Internally, try the following process to
manage some of that behavior that focuses on what we wish we offered:

1. List what makes your organization unique in your strategic
   service lines.

2. Evaluate whether the organization delivers consistently—or if it could
   do so with some work.

3. Use the list as a starting point to decide which compelling differences to
   position. Work with the internal team and leadership to determine what
   you can offer consistently that has interest for the prospective physician.

4. Once you've decided what to offer, communicate it.

In developing the regional referral strategy for East Texas Medical Center
Regional Healthcare System, VP of Strategic Planning Michael Thomas and the
organization determined that their approach was to provide a very high level
of customer service internally. "It came down to our making certain that the
people who managed the referrals were better and offered more service than
the referral sources were able to get elsewhere," he says. "And it has worked."

## What to differentiate

Some of the discussion about differentiators will feel a bit over the top. The
reason is that early programs can point to successes without such focused
methods. For programs that were early in their markets, there was less need
for this approach because the competition and the message clutter were
at a very different level. Many representatives were focused on physicians

**A Marketer's Guide to Physician Relations**

who already had some sense of loyalty. They were the group of physicians with whom the organization already had a reputation and credibility. The opportunity was to add value, provide information, encourage a relationship, and subsequently bring new business in the door.

The current situation—including the market, the competition, the expectations, and the message milieu—is vastly different. The bottom line is that we can keep business that we have earned in the past simply by offering it in the same way, as long as no one else has a better approach moving forward. If the competition is not making a compelling argument that convinces the physician there's something better, faster, easier, more considerate, and easier to access, then there's no threat of losing the business we have earned. And this is exactly why the cluttered market is taking such a toll on physician loyalty. For physicians, the number of options is overwhelming. Those organizations that already had physicians' business never really created a serious strategy to keep it. If an organization wants to grow business by taking it from a competitor, the first step is to find those compelling differences—ones that, when compared with the specific competition, make them stand apart. Look for those compelling differences in the areas of product and product delivery.

## *Product*

In the past, compelling differences were almost always at the product level. If a facility had an open heart surgery program, it assumed physicians would want to send it all heart-related cases. Now that almost all facilities have a heart program, however, or an affiliation with one and a catheterization lab, the fact that you offer the product is no longer a viable differentiator. The reality is that there are a few programs that can differentiate on product. In general, the strategy works for those organizations that have the reputation of being the first and the best to offer the service. They can leverage their reputation to add momentum to their message. For others, there's not enough substantive difference to make this an effective differentiator.

Organizations that do differentiate based purely on product need a product positioning strategy. This includes a lot of discussion about the breadth and depth of the service, and a lot of effort to detail how the patient and the referring physician benefits with outcomes. To differentiate your product in a sea of similar products requires that you go big and long and consistent, or you will not win the battle of preference and referral growth.

## Product delivery

Some organizations are working to differentiate their services based on the way the product is provided. A wonderful example is when the Labor, Delivery, Recovery and Postpartum (LDRP) programs were first introduced on maternity floors. Although they were quickly replicated, those organizations that were the first to employ the LDRP concept earned the reputation and were able to differentiate their level of patient-focused care because of a twist on how the product was delivered.

Creating innovative methods for service delivery in other areas, such as cardiac, neurosurgery, oncology, and orthopedics, is certainly possible. However, it is rarely something that is done at the suggestion of physician relations alone. It requires innovators at the leadership level, followed by implementation at the operations level. Those individuals can define what your niche area should be and then consider the possibilities.

Physician relations programs have two obligations within this environment. Their first obligation is to gather data for leadership that shows current program perceptions among that group of physicians you are targeting for growth. Once again, the ability to provide solid field intelligence is an attribute that physician relations alone can provide. Don't tell them what they want to know; tell them what they need to know. Their second obligation is that, in the event that they innovate (and especially if they innovate in the direction of your data and feedback), then there needs to be strong, consistent messaging that gets the referring physician innovators to step forward and try it. Once you get momentum on your side, shifting additional business will get easier.

## *Quality*

It was a blow for me when I discovered that the quality card can seldom stand alone. As a clinician, I valued clinical outcomes and was passionate in my belief that my hospital was the best. Years later, I realized that no physician ever chooses a hospital that has poor quality. Even with all the shifts toward more transparency, quality is really a given, lacking dramatic differences among organizations or a scandalous issue that makes the news. For physicians, the choice is rarely between a good organization and a bad one but rather between two good organizations.

The only way to differentiate on quality is to present compelling clinical data that clearly paints a picture of what you have to offer. If you believe that you have better outcomes in the key strategic service lines you are working to grow, then you have to fully develop a sales funnel that demonstrates this. The differentiating strategy is to create a good-versus-bad approach. And you need to do it without embarrassing the doctor if he or she is currently referring to another organization—the one you're positioning as bad. That can be tricky.

The best approach is to start with outliers. Begin by talking about the most complex of patients who may need different outcome levels and then begin to share data and outcomes. Provide strong rationale for the process and the approach that is used. The next time you revisit this theme with the physician, add more data and more reasons why this process is used for those very complex cases. During the third visit, you can talk about total volumes. The ability to do more means everyone benefits. Again, this requires demonstrated numbers, sometimes evidenced in length of stay or in terms of readmission rates.

If you are going to position that your quality is better, you must show it in a measurable and consistent way. Then, you need to be able to prove it in ways that make the life of the referring physician better. Certainly referring physicians like their patients to do well, but how do they benefit? And then you need to have enough quality tidbits to create an entire sales funnel based on quality.

## Patient satisfaction

Patient satisfaction is such a desirable achievement, yet it is almost never the differentiator to rely on to grow business. Why? Because physicians make

**A Marketer's Guide to Physician Relations**

their referral decisions based primarily on their perception of the best clinical outcomes, not the best patient experience. And although we know that patient satisfaction may be better at one organization than another, every facility can point to an area where it exceeds expectations. In the blur of who does what best, it becomes very difficult to cut through the confusion. Even if you are able to cut through the confusion, if the referring physician's relationship is with a specialist from another facility, this likely will not be enough to create enough differentiation to shift the referral.

The only time I suggest using patient satisfaction as a differentiator is when there is widespread discontent in the community about service issues at a key competitor. If that's the case, then create a multipronged approach that demonstrates the need for satisfaction at every level. Start by talking about physician satisfaction indicators, expand to patient and employee satisfaction indicators, and then differentiate through a discussion of why and what you understand to be ongoing strategies to sustain the momentum. Realize that the satisfaction score can be confused, rationalized, or forgotten, but the satisfaction process can position you.

### Service excellence

Positioning on service excellence can work if you look at the issue from the physician level. This one is very effort-driven and involves showing your organization is welcoming to physicians. If the level of service is going to be a differentiator, look at the growth segment and create tiered messages about service differences. Then demonstrate the impact at a professional and practice level.

For example, surgeons' number-one service differentiator is usually scheduling. As the representative works to grow the number of surgical cases, a key message will be schedule access. Following the service approach, subsequent messages will detail start times, ability to have the same staff in the room, lunch brought into the surgical waiting area for surgeons between cases, etc. The representative can create succinct messages that demonstrate the organization's efforts to provide optimal service to the surgeons. Can this make a difference? You bet it can. It assumes that you are able to deliver it consistently and also assumes your competitors can't get it together, therefore allowing you to do this.

## *First to market*

If you have the chance to communicate a first, that is a powerful way to differentiate. Years ago, I worked for an organization that had the first lithotripter for breaking up kidney stones. The momentum that we grabbed by being first and talking about it was enormous. Once you get this momentum, leverage that position of innovation to sustain the momentum. Sustaining first status for any length of time is becoming frightfully rare, so if you use this to differentiate, do it big, do it well, and hope that there is enough glow generated to sustain it.

## *Price*

In many other industries, a low-price message differentiates and draws in market share. But healthcare consumers don't want bargain-basement healthcare services unless they are paying—and even then there's significant selectivity. Although healthcare pricing has some increased application for

**A Marketer's Guide to Physician Relations**

self-pay services, the only way it really plays out as a differentiator in physician relations is in the managed care arenas. And in that regard, I do not see it as a lead differentiator. Rather, it is an obligation. If you are working to grow referrals, it makes sense to target those who can send you referrals.

# How to differentiate

Once an organization determines which clinical services to use to differentiate itself and has validated consistency in delivery and identified the unique aspects of the service that sets it apart from the others, it's time to determine how to tactically present that package to the referring physician market. One of the best ways to demonstrate this is through showcasing those who are the breadth or depth of expertise in the strategic service area that you are positioning. This is not about chest-thumping and bragging messages about the service because neither will impress. This is about crafting a role as expert for your organization by virtue of messages that demonstrate the level of expertise you have available.

### *Put a face to it*

It is very effective to harness the power of specialists and leaders. If you are able to meet with the prospective referring physician to discuss the service and begin positioning the physician's needs, you can set the stage for a meeting with the physician and one of your specialists, a clinical leader, or a member of the leadership team, depending on the physician's specific needs. With the stage set for the prospective physician, the key to differentiation is to not leave it to chance that your specialist will say the right thing. Best-practice organizations prepare the expert before the meeting. The representative should give the specialist background information on the practice, topics of interest that have come up in previous discussions, and suggestions for encouraging dialogue. A formal lecture can also work. Make certain that you know whether the specialist will use slides, and ensure that he or she knows the start and stop times of the meeting or presentation. Let the specialist know that you will follow up with the physician to learn his or her thoughts and to encourage referrals.

The expert is a strong ally to differentiate your service, especially if you have someone who is recognized. The name and face help cut through the clutter, whether he or she is recognized or not. It goes without saying, but not every specialist is a good choice. If you have someone who acts arrogant, can't relate well, or is very introverted, he or she probably isn't going to help build referral relationships. If you don't have a positive representative to present to the referring physician, find another way. Some specialists can write letters or articles, some can be part of planning, and some are good with face-to-face opportunities.

## Do it well

Anyone who works in physician relations has heard about affability, access, and ability. Referring physicians want to be respected and communicated with (affability), they want ease of entry to the hospital for themselves and their patients (access), and they want clinical competency (ability). I see these as basic requirements but not as differentiators. If the competitors are not doing it well or you do it exceptionally well, they are great value-adds. The way it works is

**A Marketer's Guide to Physician Relations**

that you position something the physicians want and you position the way you will consistently deliver it. Then you develop the message to demonstrate how it is done with respect for their needs and making access a priority, etc.

> *In our case, with tertiary pediatric referrals, there's only so much you can talk about having this kind of machine or that kind of machine; the benefits become neutral. When you're talking about competing regionally with some of the nation's top ten children's hospitals, it's all about being easy to do business with and making it as easy as possible for those physicians and their patients.*
>
> — Donna Teach, VP of marketing and public relations,
> *Nationwide Children's Hospital, Columbus, OH*

### Clinical depth

As the market becomes more sophisticated, so does the need for representatives who can really connect with the physician at a clinical level that is deeper than surface discussions. This does not mean that the representative's job is to dazzle the physician with clinical knowledge. The physician is already interested in what the representative is selling. He or she is already informed and involved.

Creating the connection is about understanding the clinical indications, knowing who would be a candidate for a certain procedure, and clearly understanding the process of admitting the patient. It's about knowing how to ask the right questions to really enhance the discussion to get the chance to position what you offer. Nor does it mean that representatives must come from a clinical background.

Representatives will most effectively differentiate themselves and the organization if they have the ability to get into a deeper dialogue at a clinical level with physicians. Many very good representatives have learned this by working in hospitals and healthcare; others are trained in the clinical aspects after they are hired. Those who have hired representatives who are great salespeople need to push the level of clinical expertise as their programs advance and their markets become more sophisticated to stay ahead in the battle for differentiation. To really grow relationships at the next level, representatives need to understand how the service is relevant for the physician's practice, including the type of patients, the type of procedures, and the frequency. The representative also must know the right questions to ask the physician to create a dialogue.

Some organizations that rely heavily on the clinical connection are using nurses in the physician realtions role. Melanie Levine, assistant director of physician relations at M. D. Anderson Cancer Center in Houston, says the center's clinical representatives are able to provide more targeted, tailored support through the use of clinical trials. This knowledge allows them to suggest those studies that are most relevant for the physicians' patients. I have worked with some outstanding nonclinical representatives who are among the best in the business at this. They step forward and make friends in the hallways with clinical staff, the service leaders, and operations team alike.

 **A Marketer's Guide to Physician Relations**

They read, they observe, and they stay focused on going back into those clinical areas to learn what's new.

## Data

Using data is an excellent way to demonstrate your position. However, data do not stand alone as a differentiator. You must define your differentiator and then use the data to demonstrate it.

Numbers sell in healthcare, both within organizations and with referring physicians. The ability to get meaningful data that can be presented in a timely manner is a chronic challenge for physician relations representatives. Yet, it is the single best tool we have to demonstrate most differences. The kind of data that is helpful is generally that which demonstrates proof of expertise, proof of outcomes, or proof that what you are selling is true. For example:

- Data that demonstrate proof of expertise can include number of cases, case mix in a service line, credentials of specialists, number of advanced cases, and special certifications.

- Data that demonstrate outcomes include mortality, morbidity, and readmit rates; returns to the OR; or complication rates. It can also include status of discharge reports and the number of patients who returned to their communities.

- Data that demonstrate you are good include door-to-balloon times for cardiac catheterization, trauma, statistics on OR turnaround times, and top 100 status.

Sometimes it is also good to have comparative data. If you are unable to do local comparisons, consider state or national averages. Once you've provided the data, clinical experts can assist by highlighting those data elements that are meaningful. It is important to sift through all the data and then create clean, easy-to-understand graphic representations of your points of differentiation.

Be strategic about how you use the data to position your expertise. Rather than dumping all the data at once, vary the presentation. Sometimes you can use information to support your talking points, while at other times it makes a good leave-behind to reinforce the discussion. Everyone in healthcare has an appreciation of outcomes, but we're all cognizant that there are so many different types of personalities that even in the world of data, it is not a one-size-fits-all application. Although I like a consistent look for all printed pieces, you can vary the presentation of the content, recognizing that some like to read more detail and some just like the pictures!

Data must be updated regularly. Nothing will get dismissed more quickly than old or slightly off-target data. If you are going to present data, it must be current and accurate, and you must have the rationale to back it up.

I once helped a client who'd done some independent survey work, which the client then asked me to present to members of the client's medical staff leader-

   **A Marketer's Guide to Physician Relations**

ship team. The sample size was too small, and there was an inaccuracy in one of the tables. The entire meeting went south very quickly—even though the rest of the data were accurate and the sample size had no relevance or impact.

When you bring data, understand the tools for gathering, the methods and impact, and when and how any survey questions were asked and answered. Often, given the way the brain of a physician works, you will be asked to defend your numbers. The more complicated, the more they will pick through the data, so keep it simple and know what you are defining.

As more and more programs enter the market, the need for differentiation will move from nice to obligatory. As with so many things, those who are proactive and have started to gather and use this data before they have to are the ones who will be seen as leaders and experts.

## Communicating differentiation

To have an impact with any approach you select to differentiate, you've got to be committed to good, strong, focused messages that advance the physician's buy-in and make the choice to refer to you a logical one. And with messaging bombarding the physician from every direction, we have to say it—and say it again and again—and we have to find multiple ways to craft the message. Every aspect of our communication needs to position this. This is why we can't do flavor-of-the-month physician relations messaging and have an impact with new business. Those who talk about a different service line each month don't get face time with physicians and don't make an impact. The product pitch is not what the physician needs. Focused messages on relevant topics with consistent messaging are essential.

Physicians have more to think about in a day than your message. Be memorable, brief, easy, interesting, and engaging. This seldom happens without some preplanning. The same holds true for the need to preplan some good questions. Take the time to think through the dialogue so you are prepared to go in any of several different directions based on the physician's responses and interests.

Here are some other considerations as you think about messages that can differentiate you:

- Physicians are caregivers. They are very interested in doing what is right for their patients. But the message and communication need to also address their needs beyond the patient experience.

- Succinct messages delivered consistently on the same topic and that add depth and breadth to the conversation are right on the money.

- Family physicians and internists are not about first-on-the-block thinking. They like to have what others have.

- If people know you for something, use that to your advantage. Help those within your organization understand the value of focus as a growth strategy. Once you get the referring physician's business, then

**A Marketer's Guide to Physician Relations**

you can begin messaging that gains expansion and more breadth. But to lure a physician in, it always works better to go with your focused area of expertise.

- Beautiful ads are not going to do it for the doctor—actually, they don't work well for the patient, either, unless there is a compelling reason to buy that is associated with it.

## Public relations

Some organizations do a great job of creating the public persona of experts through their public relations efforts. As you work to communicate with the physicians about a special area of expertise, don't forget to carry the same message into the media spotlight. Having prospective patients hear and see your organization can add to the perception of expertise and, at minimum, be a great reminder.

When you are trying to grow the relationship with the primary care physician (PCP), develop a story that talks about the PCP's diagnosis and referral and then the specialist's intervention. Early on in a new relationship, it can pay huge dividends. And although large metro newspapers are not often interested in this level of human-interest story, if you are working to grow regional referrals, the smaller papers are much more receptive.

## Custom publications

While your general approach and the areas you select to highlight stay consistent, there is a tremendous need to create messages around the topic areas

CHAPTER EIGHT

that are personalized to the physician, his or her practice, and the environment. For organizations that do a great deal of regional referral development, it's important to realize that physicians who refer from farther away are often most interested in expedient transport and consistent follow-up. On the other hand, local physicians are more interested in their own involvement, especially when other specialists who are involved. Different needs and challenges, different expectations, and careful planning of the message, the questions asked, and even the data and support tools used are all part of the positioning strategy.

## Leadership support

Those who are working to create a best-in-class model for differentiation of their organization and their relationship strategy realize that focus is again the challenge. If we try to be all things to all people, we lose the ability to create our position. It's okay to have everything. But rely on a handful of areas that differentiate you, and let the other services function as value-added benefits. In other words, they are present, they are important, and there is communication when it is of interest to the referring physician.

In my experience, this is not always easy for leaders to understand. Understand that how you grow is to stay on target with your message. When we have earned the referrals and assured the referring physicians of their wisdom in shifting that business to us, then the way we introduce other services is through a value-add strategy.

The internal message to make this happen is to say that we can't grow every service line at once by expecting the representative to pull a variety of offer-

224      © 2007 HCPro, Inc.   **A Marketer's Guide to Physician Relations**

ings from the primary care providers; it needs to be a one-at-a-time approach. It's very important to provide the rationale for differentiation, along with the cost and the impact it will have, to the senior leaders so that there is measurable reward.

Lest you think this means that we are better off with a representative who is focused on just one area, let me dispel that notion. In Chapter 3, there was ample discussion of the value of one representative who owns the relationship. I am a 100% believer in using a generalist approach—that is, having a representative who is able to discuss all aspects of the hospital. When it comes to messages and growth, it is all about selection of specialty areas and working the top two to five. The representative brings key messages to the meeting. But if the physician wants to discuss another topic, the representative should be well-versed, responsive, and open to that.

## A word about office staff

Once we have finally created differentiation to earn new referrals, the next step is to ensure that the implementation happens as promised. The office staff's understanding and willingness to give our organization a try is a critical element in success. Many staff dislike change even more than the physicians do. And although the staff is not the central decision-maker, if the staff reports glitches, we are in trouble, even with strong differentiation and best data to prove it.

As you select your approach for differentiating your product and service for the physician, take the time to create messages that will be relevant to support the transition for the office staff. For the office staff, it's about access and ease of patient communication. Craft your messages with the same effort for the staff and its needs.

At a time when everyone wants to grow their volumes and few have a solid approach to differentiation, this is the area where best-practice organizations seek to enhance their skills. The challenge is that nothing in this is glamorous— it is all hard work and very effort driven. It is also not a campaign that is implemented once. Rather, it becomes a way of doing business long term. The benefit, of course, is that there are measurable rewards in the form of new referrals, and there is internal support for the program's long-term growth. There are a few simple steps that can help remind representatives of the fundamentals for making this happen:

1. Be a good listener. Even if the representative was hired because he or she is a great talker, at the end of the day, the ability to ask good questions and to really hear the perceptions, needs, interests, and concerns of the referring physician is the differentiator.

2. Take the time to learn the products and craft the messages at the right level of depth, but with simple, easy messages. Learning is ongoing, and the healthcare delivery system is complex. Lifelong learning is more than just a phrase in the industry. It's a way of life. The best way to learn is through experts in the areas. Find your approach, and take

the time and make the effort to understand the products, how they are delivered, who does what, what tests are required, and how and when the physicians would need to be consulted.

3. Be innovative. Try new ways to cut through the clutter. Based on your target physicians and what they tell you they need, consider the possibilities and other methods for communicating your differences.

4. Stay focused. This is the greatest challenge for "can do" people. A lack of focus will insidiously take the best program off course in small, seemingly inconsequential ways until, all of a sudden, the results and measures are not what they were and there is lack of clarity. Many nice things are done and/or talked about, but they are not difference-makers.

5. Use your clinical experts. Create strategies for involving clinical experts and specialists. Put a face to the service, and use this opportunity to help them understand the role of physician relations and the importance of consistent service delivery.

6. Assure the physician of his or her wisdom. Support the physician's decision to try you with recognition of the choice and then excellent follow-up to assure the physician that the service was delivered in the way you promised.

Those who are embracing physician relations clearly understand that past success is no guarantee of future success. If you can leverage it to provide a quality that is relevant for the here and now, then there is potential. Don't assume that everyone knows you are good or what you have to offer. To paraphrase a quote I once heard that has always stuck in my mind: The greatest waste is business that goes elsewhere simply because the customer didn't know what you offer. Depend on messages that are told cleanly, clearly, succinctly, and with relevance.